Neuro-Ophthaln
Clinical Procedures

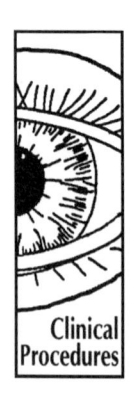

Clinical Procedures Series

Chris J. Cakanac, O.D., F.A.A.O., Series Editor

Modica PA. *Neuro-Ophthalmic System* (1999)

Schmidt EE. *Lids and Nasolacrimal System* (1997)

Cakanac CJ, Ajamian PC. *Cornea and Conjunctiva* (1996)

Johnston RL. *Retina, Vitreous, and Choroid* (1995)

Neuro-Ophthalmic System
Clinical Procedures

Patricia A. Modica, O.D.
Assistant Clinical Professor, State University of New York, State College of Optometry, New York

BUTTERWORTH HEINEMANN

Boston   Oxford   Auckland   Johannesburg   Melbourne   New Delhi

Copyright © 1999 by Butterworth–Heinemann

A member of the Reed Elsevier group

All rights reserved.

No part of this publication may be reproduced, stored in a retrieval system, or transmitted in any form or by any means, electronic, mechanical, photocopying, recording, or otherwise, without the prior written permission of the publisher.

Every effort has been made to ensure that the drug dosage schedules within this text are accurate and conform to standards accepted at time of publication. However, as treatment recommendations vary in the light of continuing research and clinical experience, the reader is advised to verify drug dosage schedules herein with information found on product information sheets. This is especially true in cases of new or infrequently used drugs.

∞ Recognizing the importance of preserving what has been written, Butterworth–Heinemann prints its books on acid-free paper whenever possible.

GLOBAL RELEAF 2000 Butterworth–Heinemann supports the efforts of American Forests and the Global ReLeaf program in its campaign for the betterment of trees, forests, and our environment.

Library of Congress Cataloging-in-Publication Data

Modica, Patricia A.
    Neuro-ophthalmic system : clinical procedures / Patricia A. Modica.
       p.   cm. -- (Clinical procedures series)
    Includes bibliographical references and index.
    ISBN 0-7506-9620-6 (alk. paper)
    1. Neuroophthalmology--Diagnosis. I. Title. II. Series.
    [DNLM: 1. Eye Diseases--diagnosis. 2. Nervous System Diseases--diagnosis. 3. Diagnosis, Differential. WW 141 M692n 1999]
    RE725.M63 1999
    617.7'15--dc21
    DNLM/DLC
    for Library of Congress   98-46226
                                                                                                             CIP

British Library Cataloguing-in-Publication Data
A catalogue record for this book is available from the British Library.

The publisher offers special discounts on bulk orders of this book.
For information, please contact:

Manager of Special Sales
Butterworth–Heinemann
225 Wildwood Avenue
Woburn, MA 01801-2041
Tel: 781-904-2500
Fax: 781-904-2620

For information on all Butterworth–Heinemann publications available, contact our World Wide Web home page at http://www.bh.com

10 9 8 7 6 5 4 3 2 1

Printed in the United States of America

Contents

	Preface	vii
	Acknowledgments	ix
	Introduction	xi
1.	Extraocular Muscle and Motility Evaluation in Acquired Strabismus	1
2.	Pupil Evaluation	35
3.	Visual Field Evaluation in Neuro-Ophthalmic Disease	69
4.	Systemic Neurologic Evaluation	111
5.	Additional Neuro-Ophthalmic Testing	133
	Index	157

Preface

Patients presenting with signs or symptoms of possible neurologic disease are common in optometric practice. The intent of this book is to provide guidelines to eye care clinicians that enable a clear, concise approach to the evaluation of patients with ocular manifestations of neurologic disease. Each chapter provides detailed instructions for neuro-ophthalmic procedures, as well as photographs and diagrams to emphasize key points. Because clues provided in the patient history play a crucial role in the differential diagnosis of neuro-ophthalmic disorders, history-taking guidelines are included to assist the clinician in the diagnostic process. Procedures are followed by interpretations and significance of abnormal results. Finally, billing and reimbursement guidelines, with appropriate International Classification of Diseases-9 and Current Procedural Terminology codes, are summarized in each chapter.

This manual is designed to enable clinicians to increase their level of comfort with complicated clinical scenarios in which benign disorders must be separated from serious conditions requiring rapid intervention. The importance of this goal becomes more significant as changes in our health care delivery system have resulted in an ever-increasing demand for eye care providers to assume greater responsibility for their patients.

P.A.M.

Acknowledgments

Special thanks go to Jonathan Stevens, O.D., for his photographic contributions. I would also like to thank my family for their encouragement and support while I worked on this project.

Introduction

The Clinical Procedures Series endeavors to provide a practical guide to common eye care procedures to the contemporary optometrist. As the role of optometry evolves, this clinical expertise is rapidly becoming a standard of competence in the profession. Divided into sections by common ocular anatomy, each volume describes how to understand, perform, and bill eye care procedures in clinical practice.

Chris J. Cakanac

1

Extraocular Muscle and Motility Evaluation in Acquired Strabismus

The complaint of diplopia implies acquired strabismus and poses a challenge due to its diagnostic complexity and neurologic implications. Because most clinicians do not encounter true paralytic strabismus on a routine basis, the level of comfort is often lacking with these cases. It is important for providers of eye care to recognize causes of ocular misalignment and differentiate true neurologic disease from benign imposters. Making accurate clinical decisions is important because of the frequently urgent nature of the disorder. Furthermore, correctly recognizing the benign nature of a condition can save the patient from expensive diagnostic studies.

Evaluating the patient with acquired strabismus consists not only of identifying the extraocular muscle (EOM) or disorder involved, but also in localizing the source of the pathology in the efferent pathway and in evaluating patients for associated systemic and neurologic disease.

Indications for pursuing a comprehensive diplopia workup include the patient who reports symptoms of diplopia, as well as the noncommunicative individual who demonstrates signs of a potential motility disturbance. Such signs include the presence of a head or face turn or tilt, closure of one eye, or a ptosis. It should also be kept in mind that patients with an acute motility disturbance may be asymptomatic if they lack binocular vision.

■ History Taking

The approach to the patient with diplopia should include a careful history. Four important questions should always be asked of all diplopia patients:

1. *Does the diplopia disappear when either eye is covered?* Diplopia from true ocular misalignment will always disappear when either eye is covered. In nearly all cases, diplopia that persists monocularly is due to a media disturbance. Such disturbances include an uncorrected refractive error, corneal or tear film abnormality or irregularity, lens changes or subluxation, and polycoria and will typically resolve with the application of a multiple pinhole occluder. In general, monocular diplopia from these causes is typically an overlapping, or "ghosting," of images rather than two distinct and separate images. Other more unusual causes of monocular diplopia include anomalous retinal correspondence in a patient with prior strabismus surgery[1] and in rare cases of cortical disease.[2,3] Although these occurrences are, in fact, unusual, they should be kept in mind in the instance where pinhole occlusion does not resolve monocular diplopia. Hysteria or malingering should also be considered when all other causes have been ruled out. Once it is determined that true ocular misalignment is present, the next three questions help to isolate the muscle(s). The hallmark of acquired strabismus is incomitance, which is defined as misalignment that varies with gaze position. Knowing where the diplopia is most apparent enables the examiner to narrow down the possibilities.

2. *Is the diplopia horizontal or vertical?* Twelve EOMs control eye movements: Eight control vertical eye movements and four control horizontal movements. Knowing whether the double vision is vertical or horizontal narrows the possibilities to eight or four muscles, respectively (Figure 1.1).

3. *Is the double vision greater at distance or near?* Double vision that is worse at distance is more likely to be caused by muscles that diverge or elevate the eyes (Figure 1.2A), whereas diplopia that is more pronounced at near is more likely to be caused by muscles that converge or depress the eyes (Figure 1.2B).

4. *Is the diplopia worse in right or left gaze?* This question helps lateralize the diplopia to muscles that have their greatest actions in right or left gaze (Figure 1.3).

After completing these questions, it is often possible for the clinician to narrow down the possibilities to the precise EOM impairment(s). The history should then be directed toward possible etiologies. For example, diplopia that occurs suddenly with little or no change suggests an ischemic or vascular etiology, whereas diplopia that shows a gradual worsening can result from Graves' orbitopathy or a compressive lesion.

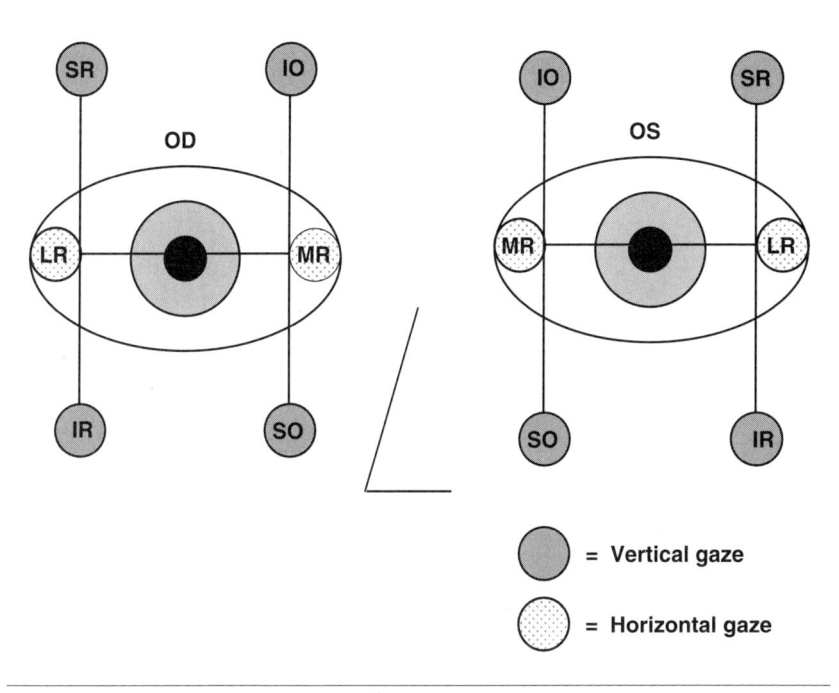

Figure 1.1 The relationship of extraocular muscles to the direction of eye movements in the diagnostic positions of gaze with vertical and horizontal movements emphasized. (LR = lateral rectus; MR = medial rectus; SR = superior rectus; IR = inferior rectus; IO = inferior oblique; SO = superior oblique.)

Diplopia from myasthenia gravis has a variable amplitude, is frequently absent after sleep, and tends to worsen later in the day. Careful questioning of the patient's past and present health status may reveal some clues regarding etiology as well. Patients should be questioned regarding a history of diabetes or its symptoms, as well as hypertension or atherosclerotic disease and giant cell arteritis, because these conditions predispose patients to infarctions of the peripheral nerve trunk. Evidence of an over- or underactive thyroid points to Graves' orbitopathy. In certain geographic locations, Lyme disease is an important cause of cranial nerve palsies. Any patient with a past history of cancer who complains of diplopia should be presumed to have metastatic disease until proven otherwise. Finally, any diplopia patient who has symptoms of fever, skin rashes, and weight loss or gain may have a related systemic condition.

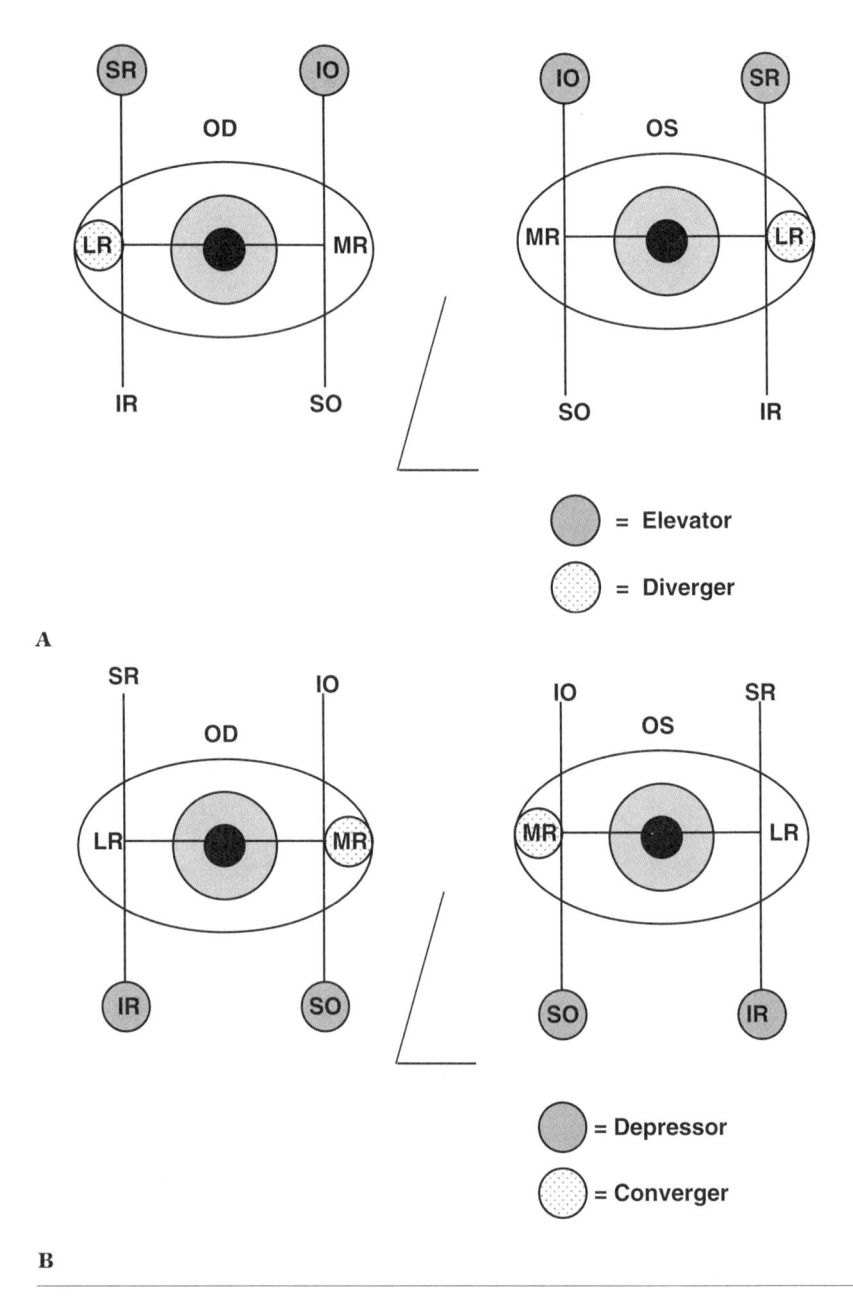

Figure 1.2 (A) The possible extraocular muscles involved when diplopia is worse at distance. (B) The possible extraocular muscles that are implicated when diplopia is worse at near. (LR = lateral rectus; MR = medial rectus; SR = superior rectus; IR = inferior rectus; IO = inferior oblique; SO = superior oblique.)

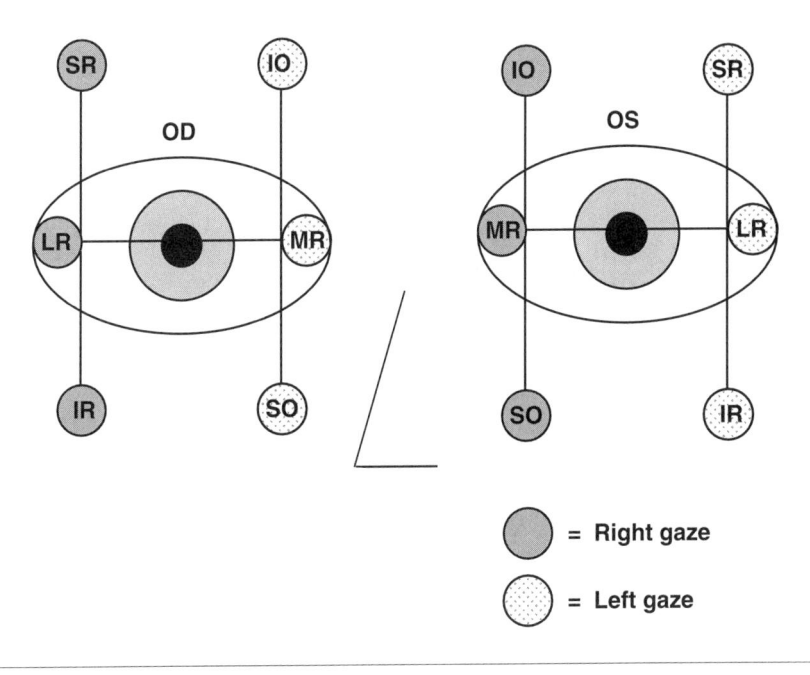

Figure 1.3 The extraocular muscles that are used in right and left gazes. (LR = lateral rectus; MR = medial rectus; SR = superior rectus; IR = inferior rectus; IO = inferior oblique; SO = superior oblique.)

The age of the patient is important in differential diagnosis, as an elderly patient is more likely to have an ischemic or vascular etiology and a younger patient is more likely to have an infectious, inflammatory, or neoplastic etiology. All these possibilities can be supported with additional medical testing or by consulting with the patient's primary physician.

Materials

Methods commonly employed in the evaluation of ocular misalignment are numerous and consist of the following types:

1. Techniques that identify the paretic muscle(s)
2. Techniques that assess the characteristics of the misalignment
3. Techniques that quantify the deviation

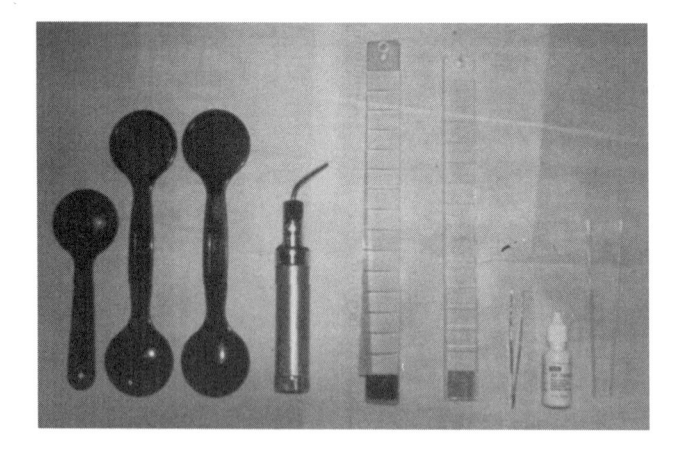

6 □ NEURO-OPHTHALMIC SYSTEM: CLINICAL PROCEDURES

Figure 1.4 Required materials for motility testing. From left to right, multiple pinhole occluder, Maddox rod, red lens, handheld light source, horizontal prism bar, vertical prism bar, toothed forceps, topical anesthetic, and cotton-tipped applicators.

The Maddox rod test, red lens test, Lancaster screen, and Parks Three-Step Test can all be used to identify the paretic muscle. Prism bars are used with some of these tests or with cover testing in different gazes to quantify misalignment. Other tests include forced ductions and evaluation of saccades, optokinetic nystagmus, ductions, the oculocephalic maneuver, and the Bell's reflex and are used to assess certain characteristics of the ocular misalignment.

The materials required for motility testing are summarized below (Figure 1.4):

> Pinhole occluder—Multiple pinhole occluders are best for confirming a non-neurologic etiology for diplopia.
> Maddox rod—Handheld Maddox rods are readily available from optical companies and should contain a red filter. The larger handheld types are best because they facilitate testing in eccentric gaze.
> Red lens—Larger, handheld varieties are better than the smaller varieties found in trial lens kits.
> Prism bars or loose prisms—Rotary prisms housed in phoropters are not recommended for incomitant misalignment because they can be used only in primary gaze.

Lancaster screen (optional)—This device, although not crucial for motility testing, has the advantage of controlling fixation so that both the primary and secondary angles of deviation can be differentiated. Although it is more likely to be found in vision training practices, it has the added advantages of both qualifying and quantifying the deviation, as well as easy application by office technicians or assistants.

Handheld light—This is used as a fixation device and it also creates a corneal reflex, which can be useful in detecting smaller deviations.

Toothed forceps—When forced-duction testing is indicated, these are used to grasp the EOM insertion at the anterior sclera to manually move the eye.

Cotton-tipped applicators—As an alternate to the toothed forceps, these can be used to manipulate the eye in forced-duction testing.

Topical anesthetic—Forced-duction testing with toothed forceps may require the use of 10% topical cocaine solution. If cotton-tipped applicators are being used, either proparacaine 0.50% or tetracaine 0.50% is needed.

Test Performance

■ Corneal Reflex Tests

In uncooperative or unresponsive patients, observation of the corneal reflections from a handheld light often provides useful information regarding ocular alignment. The subject fixates on a light held at 50 cm. With the Hirschberg test, the examiner estimates the displacement of the corneal reflex relative to the position in the fellow eye (Figure 1.5). Each millimeter of displacement corresponds to 22 prism diopters (at 33 cm, each millimeter of displacement corresponds to 15 prism diopters of misalignment). The Krimsky test involves the use of prisms to neutralize the misalignment. A disadvantage to the use of corneal reflex tests is that small amounts of misalignment are difficult to detect. In cases of paralytic strabismus, the displacement of the corneal reflexes is made more obvious as the eye fixates in the direction of the limitation.

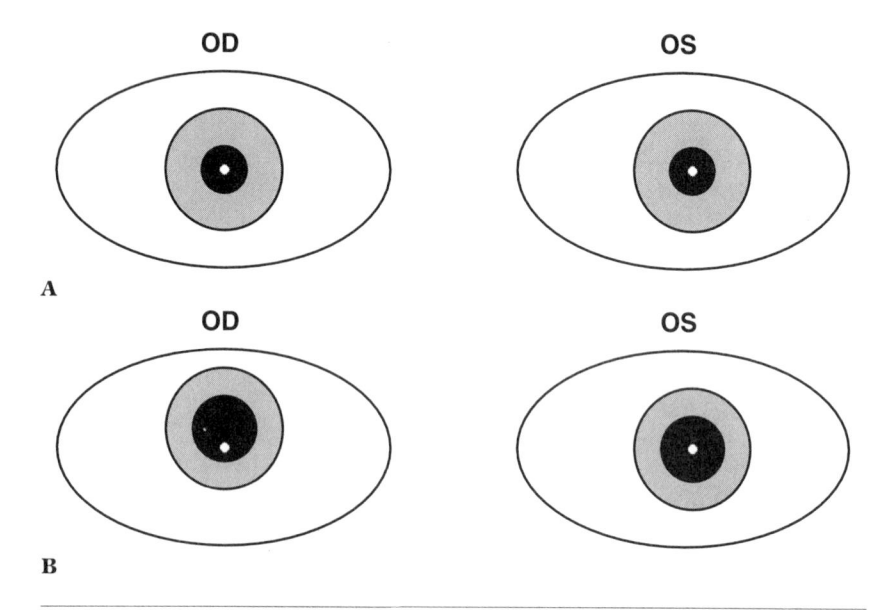

Figure 1.5 (A) The corneal reflexes in a patient without ocular misalignment. (B) The corneal reflexes in a patient with a right hypertropia. Note the downward displacement of the corneal reflex in the right eye.

■ Prism and Cover Testing

Prism and cover testing is another objective test of ocular misalignment. By alternately occluding each eye, the direction of horizontal and/or vertical eye movement on refixation alerts the examiner to the nature of the misalignment. The movement can be quantified by neutralization with a prism bar or loose prisms. Comitance can be assessed by repeating the process in the seven diagnostic positions of gaze (Figure 1.6).

■ Maddox Rod

The Maddox rod consists of a series of transparent cylinders typically with a red filter. The cylinders and filter create a red streak when the patient observes a fixation light while looking through it. A handheld model with

Figure 1.6
The seven diagnostic positions of gaze and their corresponding extraocular muscles. Observation of ocular motility in these positions enables the examiner to detect limitations in individual extraocular muscles. By holding a fixation target 40 cm from the patient, alignment is noted first in primary gaze. The eccentric positions are achieved by moving the fixation target approximately 30 degrees from fixation into the appropriate positions. (RSO = right superior oblique; LIO = left inferior oblique; RLR = right lateral rectus; LMR = left medial rectus; LSO = left superior oblique; RIR = right inferior rectus; LSR = left superior rectus; RIO = right inferior oblique; LLR = left lateral rectus; RMR = right medial rectus; RSO = right superior oblique; LIR = left inferior rectus.)

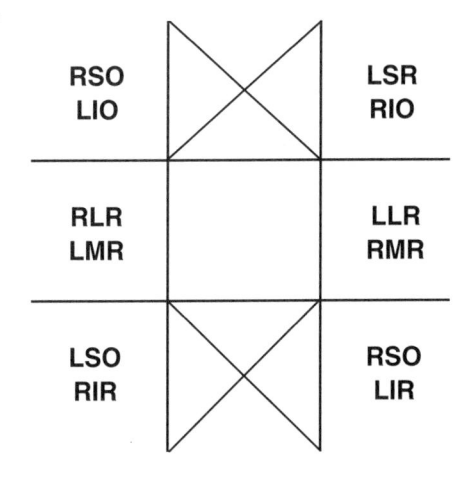

RSO LIO		LSR RIO
RLR LMR		LLR RMR
LSO RIR		RSO LIR

a red filter is best for evaluating paralytic or noncomitant strabismus. By convention, the rod is always placed in front of the right eye. With the rods oriented vertically, the patient will observe a horizontal red streak while fixating a penlight, allowing observation of vertical deviations (Figure 1.7). Horizontal orientation of the rods results in a vertical red streak, allowing qualification of horizontal misalignment (Figure 1.8). Positioning the fixation light in the diagnostic positions of gaze allows observation of comitancy. By the clinician placing the appropriate prism before an eye to neutralize the defect, the magnitude of the deviation can be measured. Findings are recorded in the seven diagnostic positions as shown in Figure 1.9.

The Maddox rod also has an important use when there is a torsional component to the misalignment. This occurs only when there is involvement of one of the cyclovertical muscles and is most important with paresis or paralysis of one of the oblique muscles. A cyclodeviation is apparent when the patient experiences tilting of one of the diplopic images. The double Maddox rod test uses two Maddox rods: One is placed before each

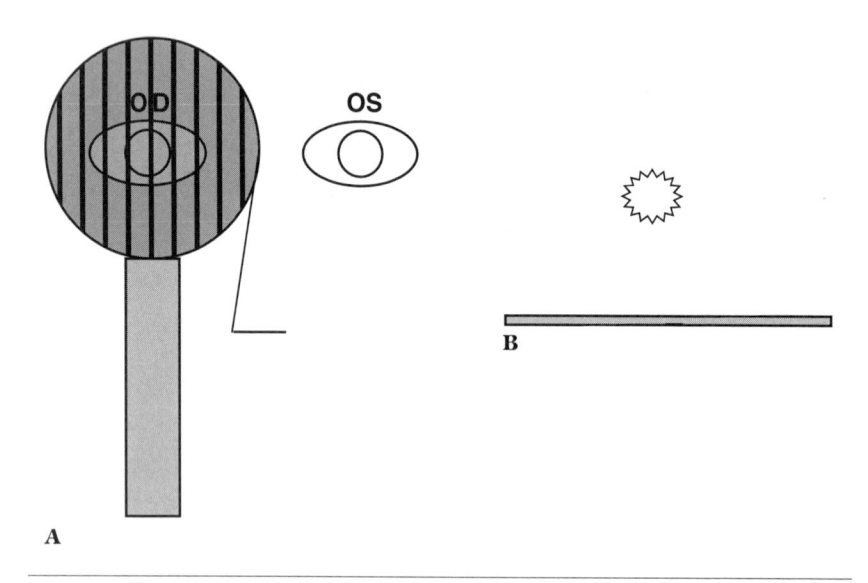

Figure 1.7 With the Maddox rod oriented vertically (A), a horizontal red streak is produced when the patient fixates a penlight (B). The red streak is seen by the right eye while a white light is seen by the left eye. The distance between the two represents the degree of vertical misalignment. The higher eye sees the lower image; therefore, the above example represents a right hypertropia.

eye. The rods are positioned vertically so that the patient sees two horizontal lines, one above the other. If a cyclodeviation is present, one of the streaks seen by the patient will be tilted. The patient is then instructed to straighten the tilted streak. By using a trial frame, the amount of cyclodeviation can be quantified in degrees (Figure 1.10). Excyclodeviations result from paresis of superior rectus and superior oblique muscles, whereas incyclodeviations result from paresis of inferior oblique and inferior rectus muscles. Cyclodeviations are best observed in the oblique muscles on adduction and on the rectus muscles on abduction.

■ Red Lens Test

Like the Maddox rod test, the red lens test employs the use of dissimilar images. A red lens is placed in front of the right eye while the patient fixates a handheld light. If fusion is present, the two lights will be superim-

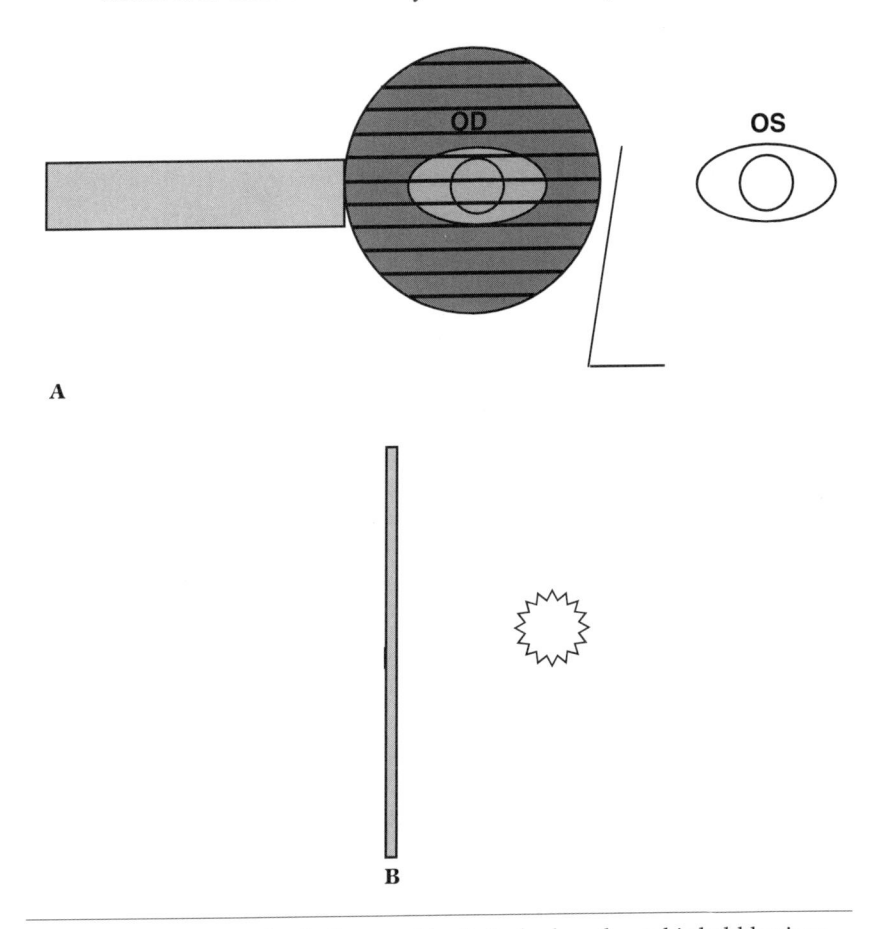

Figure 1.8 Horizontal misalignment is elicited when the rod is held horizontally (A). When the patient notices the red streak to the left of the light (B), the diplopia is crossed corresponding to an exotropia. If the streak is positioned to the right of the light, the deviation is uncrossed and the patient is esotropic.

posed. When misalignment is apparent, two lights are seen by the patient. A red light is observed with the right eye and a white light is observed with the left eye. The patient describes the relationship of the two lights in the diagnostic positions of gaze. The eye with the paretic muscle can be identified as the one that sees the more distally located image (Figure 1.11).

12 □ NEURO-OPHTHALMIC SYSTEM: CLINICAL PROCEDURES

	ortho	ortho	2 RH	
Patient's right	1 RH	5 RH	10 RH	Patient's left
	3 RH	10 RH	15 RH	

Figure 1.9 Sample recordings of vertical deviations produced by a right superior oblique palsy on Maddox rod testing. The examiner records findings in the same positions noted as they are taken. The left side of the diagram represents the patient's right gaze. (RH = right hypertropic; ortho = orthotropic.)

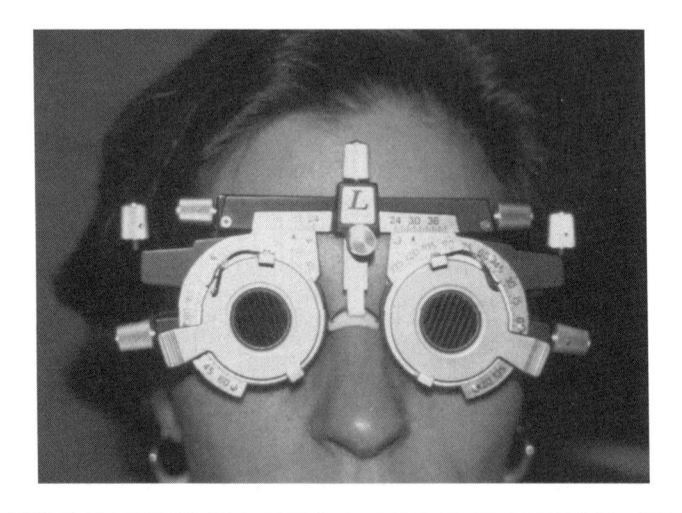

Figure 1.10 Measuring cyclorotations with Maddox rods mounted in a trial frame. The patient rotates the cylinders in the frame until they are horizontal and parallel and the degree of rotation translates to the degree of cyclodeviation. The above diagram represents excyclotorsion.

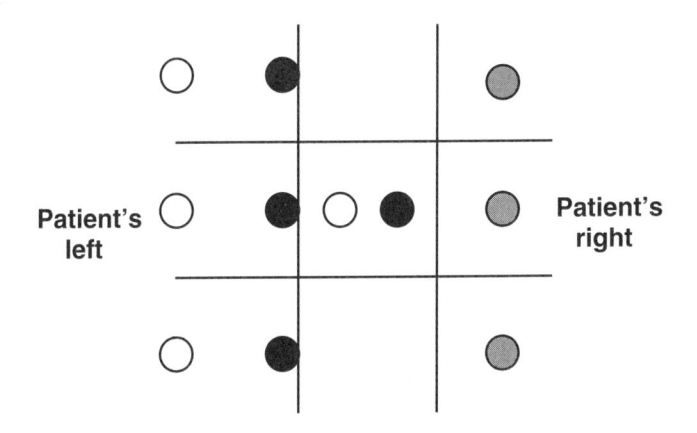

Figure 1.11 Red lens findings as a patient with a left abduction deficit sees them. This represents uncrossed, horizontal misalignment. In this case, the more distally located image is the white image; therefore, the left eye has the paretic muscle. (Black dots = red light; white dots = white light; gray dots = fusion.)

■ Lancaster Red-Green Test

Introduced by Lancaster in 1959,[4] the Lancaster red-green test uses the principle of dissimilar targets. The Lancaster screen is a shade screen, much like a white window shade, that can be rolled up when not in use. It is made up of a series of lines that form a grid of 7-cm boxes. Each box on the grid is calibrated in prism diopters so that when the patient is positioned at 2 m, each box represents 5 prism diopters. The patient wears red-green spectacles with the red filter before the right eye. The patient is given a flashlight that projects a green target while the examiner holds a red light. The room is darkened so that each eye sees a different target. The patient sees his or her green light with the right eye and the examiner's red light with the left eye. The examiner projects his or her red target onto the screen in one of the diagnostic positions of gaze, which are marked on the screen. The patient then superimposes his or her light on top of the examiner's. In the case of ocular misalignment, the patient's light will actually be located some distance away on the screen. The distance between the two lights represents the degree of misalignment. Because the squares are calibrated, the deviation can be recorded directly in prism diopters. By repeating the process in the diagnostic positions of gaze, the paretic muscle can be identified. Incomitance is

LEFT FIELD   **RIGHT FIELD**

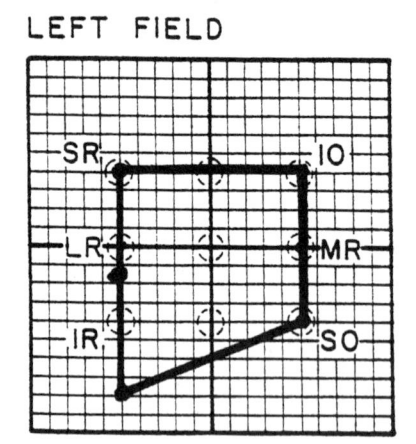

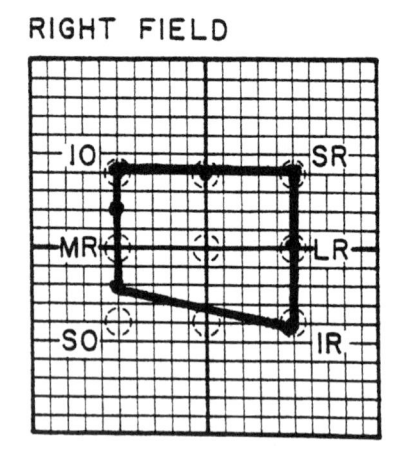

Figure 1.12 Lancaster results are recorded on a miniature version of the screen that can be placed in the chart for future reference. This example shows an underaction of the right superior oblique when the left eye fixates (right field) and an overaction of the yoked left inferior rectus when the right eye fixates (left field). (SR = superior rectus; LR = lateral rectus; IR = inferior rectus; IO = inferior oblique; MR = medial rectus; SO = superior oblique.)

readily detected by observing variations in magnitude in the different positions. The flashlights can be switched at this point, and the sequence repeated to determine the secondary angle of deviation, which reflects fixation with the paretic eye. Results are transferred to a miniature version of the screen, which can be placed in the chart for future reference (Figure 1.12).

Although the Lancaster screen is more often used by optometrists in strabismic practice, the Lancaster red-green test has perhaps its greatest value in paralytic strabismus.[1] It has the advantages of being faster because it identifies and quantifies the deviation at the same time and is easily performed by a technician or office assistant. This is especially beneficial when multiple muscles are involved. In addition, because the test distance is fixed and the squares are calibrated, it is more accurate and repeatable than the Maddox rod and red lens tests. One important aspect of the test is that it controls fixation so that the patient cannot alternate fixation from the paretic to the nonparetic eye. Finally, the test is easy for the patient to understand and for the examiner to interpret.

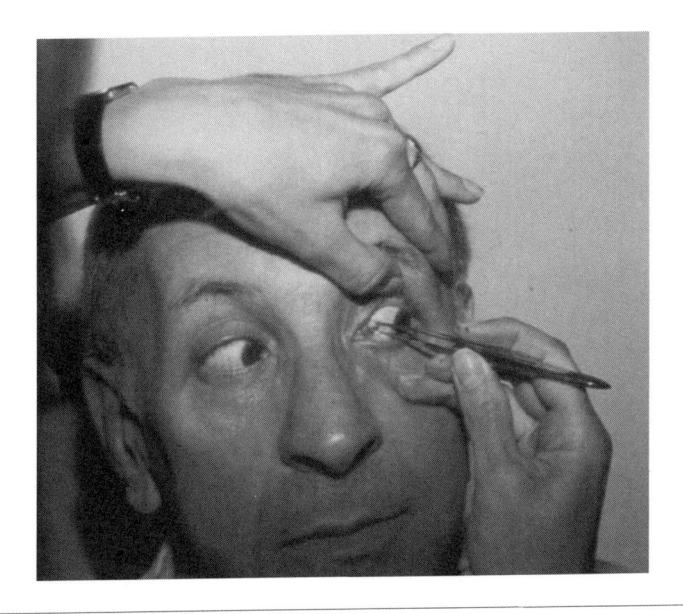

Figure 1.13 A toothed forceps is used to grasp the extraocular muscle approximately 5 mm from the limbus.

■ Forced Ductions

Forced-duction testing is essential in differentiating ocular misalignment secondary to paralytic strabismus from the misalignment caused by mechanical restriction of a muscle as seen in Graves' orbitopathy and inflammatory disease, traumatic entrapment, or structural lesions. Forced ductions can be assessed in several ways, including techniques using toothed forceps or a cotton-tipped applicator.

Forced Duction with Toothed Forceps

Proparacaine is (or tetracaine) instilled into the cul-de-sac of the eye to be tested. Additionally, a cotton-tipped applicator soaked in proparacaine or 10% cocaine is held over the insertion of the rectus muscle 5 mm posterior to the limbus for approximately 30 seconds. Conjunctiva and fascia of Tenon are grasped with a toothed forceps at the EOM insertion opposite the quadrant where the eye is to be rotated (Figure 1.13). The patient is instructed to attempt fixation in the direction of the restriction while the examiner attempts to manually pull the eye in the same direction.

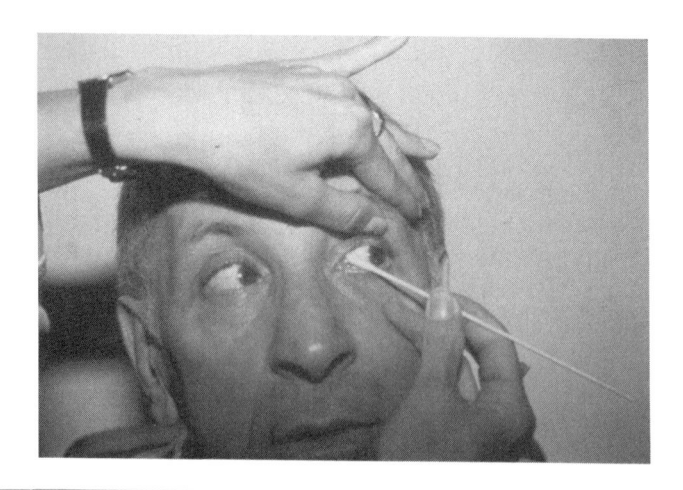

Figure 1.14 Modified forced ductions using a cotton-tipped applicator. The examiner attempts to push the eye into the direction of the restricted movement.

Mechanical restriction is confirmed by resistance to movement. The procedure should be repeated on the fellow eye to compare the range of motion. Although the procedure is generally safe, subconjunctival hemorrhage will often occur even when the technique is properly performed.

Forced Duction Using a Cotton-Tipped Applicator

Topical proparacaine or tetracaine is instilled into the cul-de-sac of the eye to be tested. The patient is then instructed to look into the direction of the muscle restriction while the examiner manually attempts to push the eye with a cotton-tipped applicator positioned just posterior to the limbus on the side opposite the direction in which the eye is to be rotated (Figure 1.14). Resistance to movement constitutes a positive response.

Although the use of a sterile, cotton-tipped applicator is less traumatic to the eye than the application of toothed forceps, there is a greater likelihood that the applicator will slip and skid over the cornea, resulting in a corneal abrasion. Furthermore, because the eye is pushed rather than pulled as with forceps, there is a greater likelihood that the globe will be displaced backward to cause a false-positive result.

Identifying Paretic Muscles

Identification of the involved muscle in the patient with diplopia involves a clear understanding of EOM function. In each eye, there are six EOMs, two of which control horizontal eye movements and four of which control cyclovertical eye movements.

■ Horizontal Misalignment

Because there are only two muscles in each eye that control horizontal eye movements, patients complaining of horizontal diplopia are easiest to address. When a patient complains of horizontal diplopia, four possible muscles may be involved: the right and left lateral recti and the right and left medial recti. By noting whether the diplopia is greater in right or left gaze, the possibilities are narrowed down to two (Figure 1.15). An example would be a patient with horizontal diplopia from a right sixth nerve palsy. If the patient reports that the horizontal diplopia is greater in right gaze, the possibilities are narrowed down to the left medial rectus muscle or the left lateral rectus muscle. If the paresis is profound, the limitation is readily observed on version testing. If it is not, however, the examiner can be aided by the use of the Maddox rod or red lens test. If the diplopia is crossed on right gaze, it represents an exotropia that would implicate the left medial rectus. In this case, the patient would see the white light to the right. The white light would also be more distally, further implicating the left eye. If the diplopia is uncrossed, it represents an esotropia that would implicate the right lateral rectus (Figure 1.16).

■ Vertical Misalignment

Patients reporting vertical diplopia pose a greater challenge to the examiner, not only because there are more possibilities, but also because the actions of the cyclovertical muscles are more complex. When the mis-

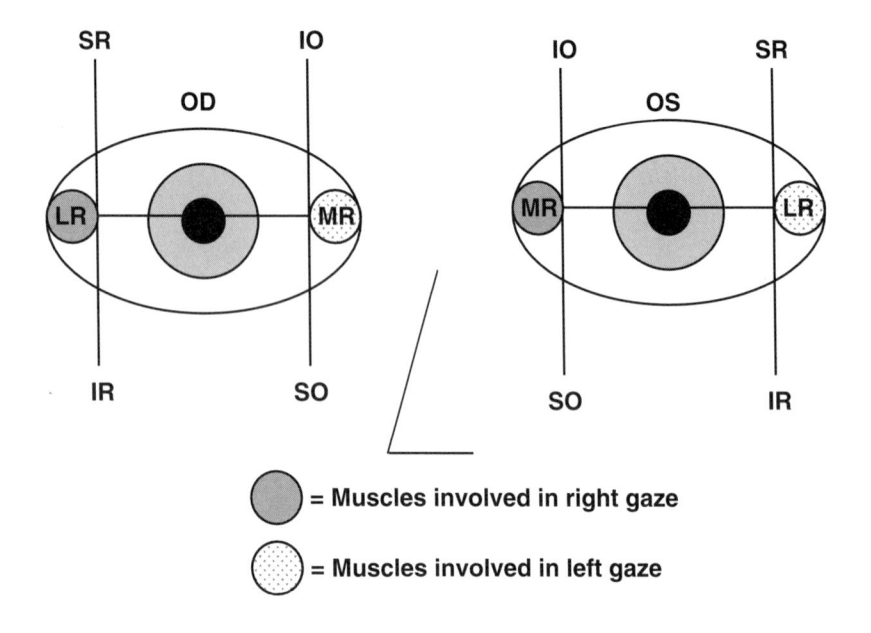

Figure 1.15 A patient complaining of horizontal diplopia has four possible muscle limitations consisting of the medial and lateral rectus muscles of each eye. If the diplopia is worse in right gaze, the possibilities are narrowed down to the right lateral rectus and right medial rectus. (LR = lateral rectus; MR = medial rectus; SR = superior rectus; IR = inferior rectus; IO = inferior oblique; SO = superior oblique.)

alignment is caused by involvement of a single cyclovertical muscle, the Parks Three-Step Test[5] can be used to identify the paretic muscle.

■ Parks Three-Step Test

Step 1 of Parks Three-Step Test determines which eye is higher in the primary position. This narrows the possibilities from eight to four. If, for example, there is a right hypertropia in primary gaze, the problem can be narrowed to the depressors of the right eye or the elevators in the left eye (Figure 1.17).

The hypertropic eye is identified by the alternate cover test or by observation of the corneal reflexes. If the misalignment is difficult to observe, a Maddox rod oriented vertically over the right eye identifies the

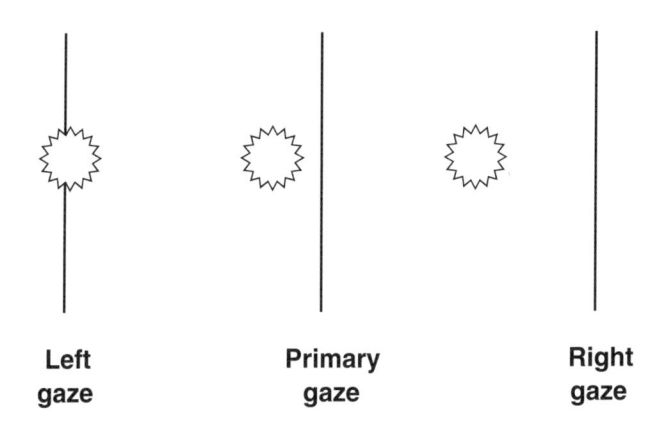

Figure 1.16 If the misalignment is not readily observed, dissociation with a Maddox rod is used to confirm the limited extraocular muscle. The above Maddox rod findings are shown from the patient's perspective. In primary gaze, misalignment is present. Because it is uncrossed, it represents an esotropia that would correspond to an abduction deficit. Note that this misalignment is incomitant and increases in right gaze.

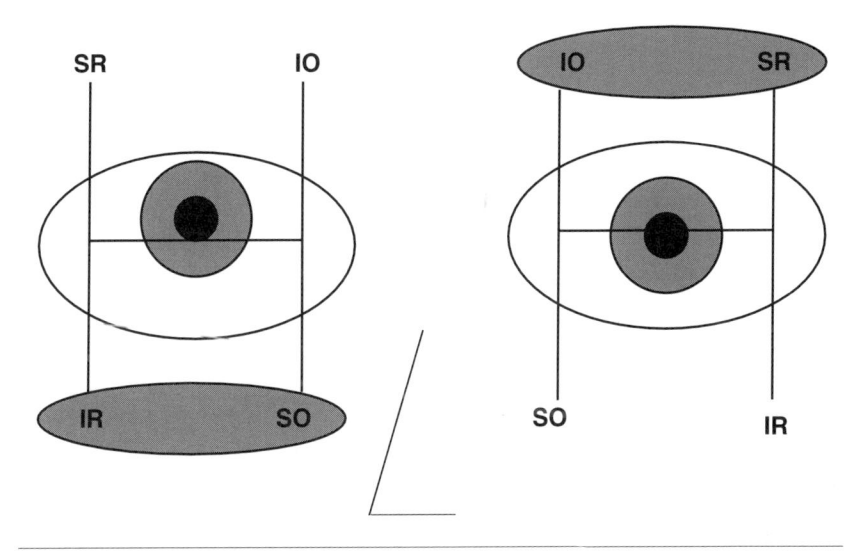

Figure 1.17 A patient with a right hypertropia. The shaded areas highlight the potential muscles involved. (SR = superior rectus; IR = inferior rectus; IO = inferior oblique; SO = superior oblique.)

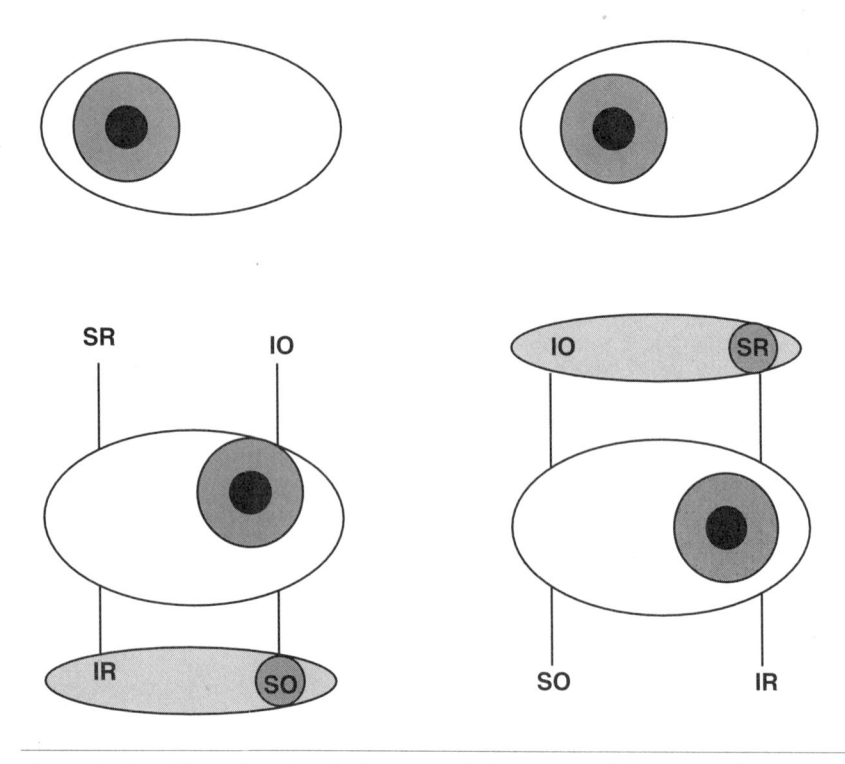

Figure 1.18 Observing that the hypertropia is worse on left gaze further narrows the possibilities to those muscles that have their greatest action in left gaze—that is, the right superior oblique and left superior rectus. (SR = superior rectus; IR = inferior rectus; IO = inferior oblique; SO = superior oblique.)

hypertropic eye. On Maddox rod testing, the higher eye sees the lower image so that in the case of a right hypertropia, the red streak is positioned lower than the white light.

Step 2 compares the amount of deviation in right and left gaze. This step further narrows the choices to two possibilities. Using the example of a right hypertropia, if the deviation is minimal on right gaze and increases on left gaze, the suspicion falls on the remaining muscles which have their greatest action in left gaze. These are identified as the right superior oblique and the right superior rectus (Figure 1.18).

Step 3 is the Bielschowsky head-tilting test. At this point, the remaining two muscles are always in different eyes. Furthermore, both muscles are either intortors or extortors, and never one of each. The third step compares the hypertropia in right and left head tilt.[6] Using the same example of a right hypertropia that increases in left gaze, comparing the hypertropia on right and left head tilts narrows the possibilities to one. Because both of these muscles are intortors, the ability of either eye to intort will be compared. The intorting action of the right superior oblique muscle is challenged on right head tilt, and the intorting action of the left superior rectus is challenged on left head tilt. If the hypertropia increases on right tilt, the right superior oblique is the final choice. On right head tilt, the right eye must intort, calling on the right superior rectus and right superior oblique. When these two muscles intort, their opposite vertical actions will cancel each other out, resulting in a torsional movement without elevation or depression. The same applies to extorsion of the inferior oblique and inferior rectus in the fellow eye. If the hypertropia increases in right tilt, the right superior oblique is implicated. If this muscle is paretic, it cannot accomplish its job of intorting the eye in response to the head tilt. Intorsion must therefore be accomplished mainly by the right superior rectus muscle whose vertical action is elevation. If the superior oblique muscle is paretic, the elevation of the superior rectus goes unopposed, and the final result is a hypertropia on right head tilt.

Interpretation

■ Third Nerve Palsy

The third cranial nerve innervates multiple EOMs, and limitations from third nerve palsy will therefore occur in multiple positions of gaze. Patients experience diplopia, which has both a horizontal and vertical component, and is apparent at both distance and near. In a complete third nerve palsy, profound ptosis is present, and the eye will be positioned down and out. The pupil may be dilated and poorly responsive, or it may be spared. The former is a neurosurgical emergency that implies a posterior communicating artery aneurysm. Motility evaluation demonstrates EOM limitations in superolateral and superomedial gaze due to involvement of the superior rectus and inferior oblique muscles, respectively. Adduction deficit is present due to medial rectus involvement. Downgaze limitations are in the direction of the inferior oblique muscle. In attempted gaze down and inward, the eye will intort due to a normally functioning superior oblique muscle. This may be seen with

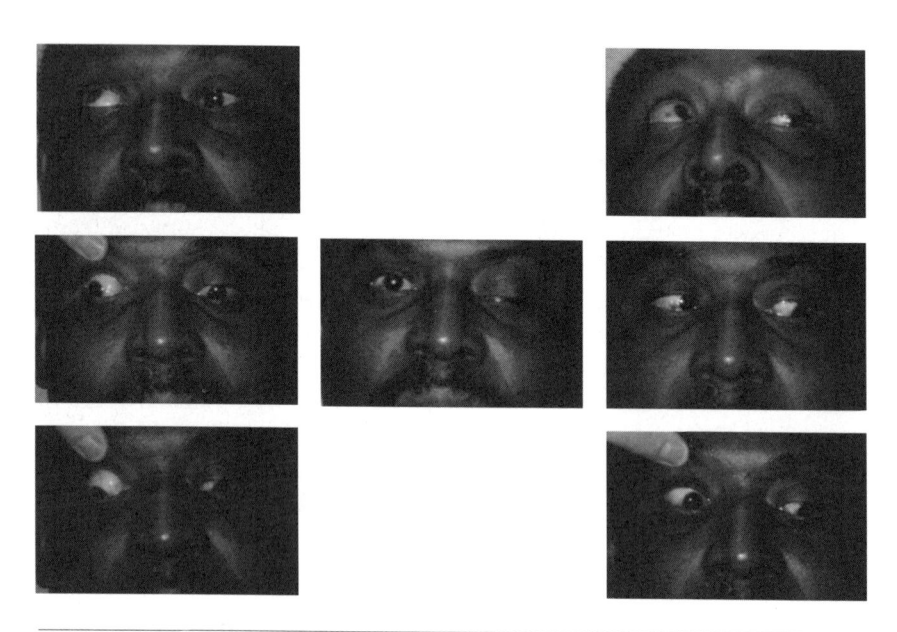

Figure 1.19 Summary of the motility findings in third nerve palsy.

careful observation. The motility findings seen in third nerve palsy are summarized in Figure 1.19. Because of multiple EOM involvement, the Lancaster screen provides the easiest means of quantifying the degree of limitation. If this is not available, red lens dissociation allows identification of the motility pattern, which can be quantified with both horizontal and vertical prism.

■ Fourth Nerve Palsy

The fourth cranial nerve or trochlear nerve innervates the superior oblique muscle. The primary action of the superior oblique muscle is depression, and the muscle is a pure depressor when the eye is adducted. The superior oblique muscle is also the primary intorter of the eye. The characteristic motility pattern of a fourth nerve palsy is an ipsilateral hypertropia that increases on contralateral gaze and ipsilateral head tilt. Patients typically report vertical diplopia that is most apparent when reading. In many cases, an observable head tilt to compensate for the vertical misalignment is observed (Figure 1.20). Often a horizontal component is present, due to an

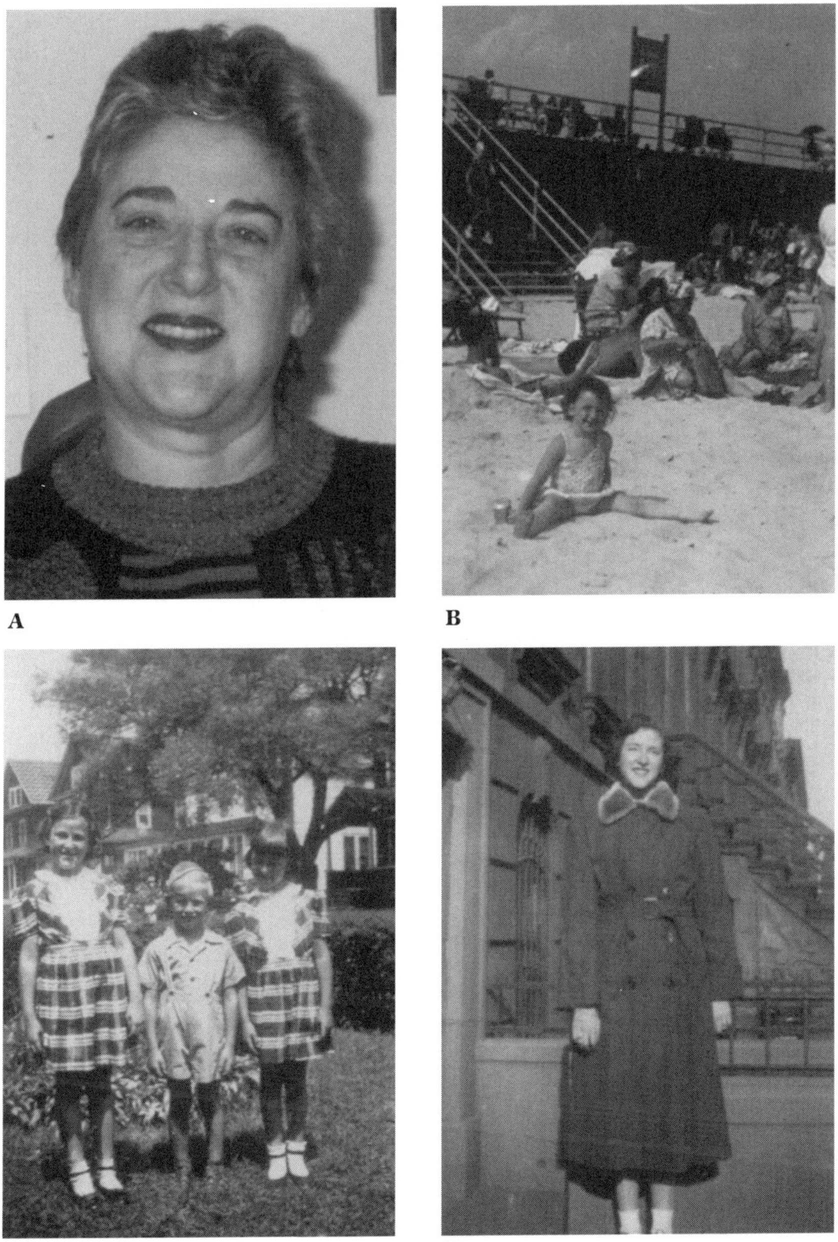

A B C D

Figure 1.20 A patient with a long-standing fourth nerve palsy demonstrating a habitual left head tilt (A). Old photographs (B–D) show that the head tilt is long-standing.

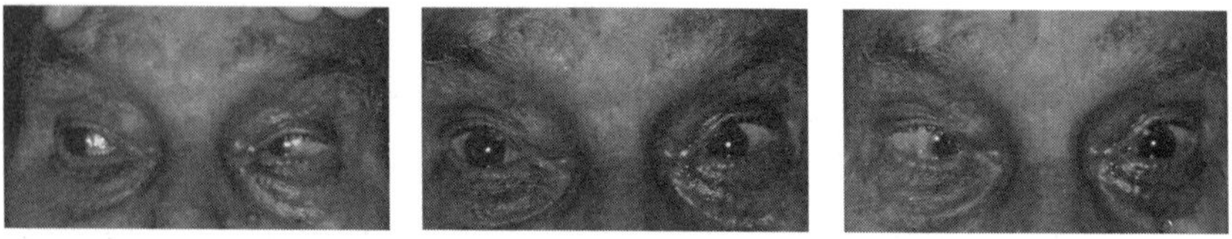

Figure 1.21 Motility pattern in a patient with a left sixth nerve palsy. (A) Right gaze. (B) Primary gaze. (C) Left gaze. Note the abduction deficit on left gaze.

overlying lateral phoria. In addition to the vertical misalignment, patients frequently report tilting of one of the diplopic images. This occurs due to the loss of intorsion of the paretic superior oblique muscle.

■ Sixth Nerve Palsy

The sixth cranial nerve, or abducens nerve, innervates the lateral rectus muscle, whose only action is abduction of the eye. Therefore, patients with sixth nerve palsy will demonstrate an abduction deficit and report horizontal diplopia, which is most apparent on ipsilateral gaze (Figure 1.21). Because the lateral rectus muscle is used to diverge the eyes, the diplopia is also most apparent at distance and improves at near. On Maddox rod or red lens testing, the patient reports uncrossed diplopia greater on ipsilateral gaze (see Figure 1.16). Saccadic velocity gives important information regarding paralysis of the lateral rectus muscle.[7] With abducens paralysis, the lateral rectus muscle cannot move the eye on attempted abduction. Instead, there is only relaxation of the medial rectus muscle, resulting in a passive drift of the eye toward the midline. This is readily observed clinically by having patients fixate back and forth at two fingers held so that the affected eye moves from the adducted position and primary gaze alternately. An optokinetic stimulus can be used to elicit rapid, repetitive saccades as well.

■ Graves' Ophthalmopathy

Motility disturbances and other eye findings are common in patients with primary autoimmune thyroid disease. In most cases, ophthalmic manifes-

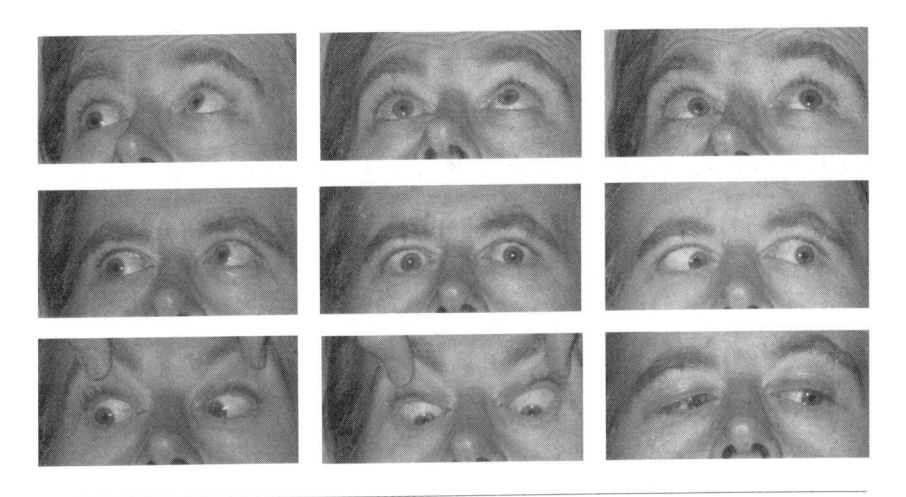

Figure 1.22 Motility findings in a patient with Graves' orbitopathy. Note restrictions in upgaze and abduction, as well as eyelid retraction in primary gaze.

tations appear within 18 months of the appearance of thyroid disease[8] but may also precede or be unassociated with clinical or biochemical evidence of thyroid dysfunction (euthyroid Graves'). Because the ocular manifestations follow a different clinical course than the thyroid dysfunction and may even occur in isolation, the terms *Graves' ophthalmopathy* and *Graves' orbitopathy* are more appropriate than the traditionally used *thyroid* or *dysthyroid ophthalmopathy*.

Although the precise mechanism of Graves' orbitopathy is not known, it is understood that the process is driven by hormonal and autoimmune processes that lead to accumulation of mucopolysaccharides (hyaluronic acid) within the EOMs and orbital fat. Together with interstitial edema and inflammatory cell reaction, there is an increase in orbital content, as well as several other ocular manifestations.

Motility disturbances in Graves' orbitopathy are the result of infiltration and inflammation within the EOMs. The result is EOM enlargement with mechanical restriction of gaze in the opposite field of action of the infiltrated muscle (Figure 1.22). Therefore, with infiltration of the medial rectus, an abduction deficit results that is often mistaken for a sixth nerve palsy. The key test for the diagnosis of this mechanical restriction is forced-duction testing, which will be positive. Comparison of intraocular pressure (IOP) measurements in both primary gaze and on attempted gaze into the direction of the restriction often provides useful information regarding the nature of EOM limitation. If the IOP increases by 5 mm Hg or more on attempted gaze into the restricted field, mechanical restriction is confirmed.[9] Another observation that will help differentiate the motility disturbance seen in Graves' from other neuro-ophthalmic disorders is the frequent presence of enlarged and hyperemic EOM insertions that can be seen through the conjunctiva. Often the conjunctival vasculature is engorged in these areas as well (Color Plate 1). The presence of additional features of Graves' orbitopathy is crucial to making an accurate diagnosis. The earliest and most common finding is eyelid retraction. Although the eyelid retraction seen in hyperthyroid disorders may result from increased sympathetic tone, the lid retraction most commonly associated with Graves' is due to mechanical restriction of the levator secondary to adhesion of the levator muscle to fixed ocular tissues.[10,11] Mechanical restriction of the levator is apparent when the examiner grasps the lid at the lashes and observes resistance on attempt to manually lower the lid. This "eyelid forced-duction test" is helpful in the differential diagnosis of other causes of eyelid retraction as is the observance of lid lag on downgaze (Graefe's sign).

Other features of Graves' orbitopathy include exophthalmos and eyelid edema, which are the result of infiltration, inflammation, and edema of the orbital contents. Exophthalmos is rarely an isolated finding and often results in exposure keratitis, especially because it is typically accompanied by lid retraction. A rare manifestation of Graves' orbitopathy is the occurrence of a compressive optic neuropathy due to crowding of the orbital contents at the orbital apex. Although this finding occurs in less than 5% of Graves' orbitopathy patients,[12] it can lead to devastating visual loss if not treated. Signs of compressive optic neuropathy include hyperemia and/or swelling of the disc, optic nerve pallor, and signs of optic nerve dysfunction (vision loss, afferent pupillary defect, dyschromatopsia, and visual field defects).

■ Internuclear Ophthalmoplegia

The combination of an adduction deficit with a contralateral abducting nystagmus is characteristic of internuclear ophthalmoplegia (INO). It is caused by a unilateral lesion of the medial longitudinal fasciculus (MLF) anywhere along its connections between the sixth and third nerve nuclei in the pons or midbrain (Figure 1.23). A lesion of the right MLF results in

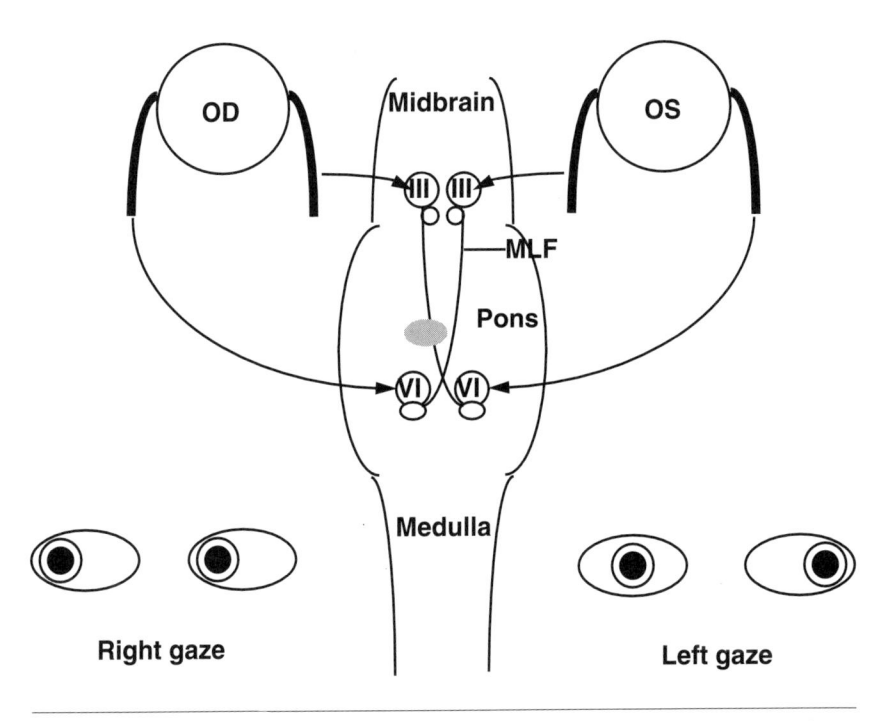

Figure 1.23 Ventral view of brain stem connections between the third and sixth nerve nuclei via the medial longitudinal fasciculus (MLF). A lesion of the right MLF results in right abduction deficit, which is most apparent on attempted left gaze.

a right adduction deficit and a left beating abducting nystagmus on attempted left gaze. The opposite occurs in a left MLF lesion. The abducting nystagmus is not always present. Convergence may be absent or spared. If convergence is absent, the location of the lesion is in the mesencephalon. If it is spared, the lesion is in the pons. Because the MLF is a midline structure, it is possible to lesion both sides simultaneously. The result of a bilateral lesion is a bilateral INO. The same localizing rules apply.

As with lateral rectus palsies, the INOs will also exhibit a slowed adducting saccade in the direction of the adduction deficit. In fact, INOs may show only a slowed adduction saccade with otherwise normal adduction on versions testing.

Unilateral or bilateral INO in a young adult is most likely due to demyelinating disease. In those older than 50, it is most likely due to brain stem infarction. INO is often accompanied by upbeating nystagmus or skew deviation. Skew deviation is a vertical misalignment of the eyes which may be comitant or incomitant. The misalignment cannot be isolated to a single EOM, and no torsional component is present. Skew deviations are the result of a disturbance of prenuclear inputs to the nuclei controlling vertical alignment of the eyes.[13]

■ Myasthenia Gravis

Myasthenia gravis is a neuromuscular disorder characterized by weakness and fatigue of voluntary muscle. The etiology is autoimmune, and in most cases, it appears that antibodies are produced that interfere with neuromuscular transmission by reducing the number of acetylcholine receptors at the postsynaptic neuromuscular junction.[14] The disorder may be apparent in extraocular, bulbar, and/or limb muscles. When the disease is confined to the extraocular, levator, and orbicularis muscles, it is referred to as *ocular myasthenia gravis*. Ptosis and EOM involvement are the most common ocular manifestations (Figure 1.24). The diagnosis of myasthenia gravis is very often an elusive one because it can mimic any motility disturbance. In many instances, it is only after repeated evaluation that the correct diagnosis is made as the motility pattern takes on a different look. In patients with ocular myasthenia, 90% have ptosis and extraocular involvement, 25% have orbicularis weakness, and 10% have ptosis alone.[15] The key to diagnosing myasthenia gravis is to understand that the muscle weakness is variable, improves with rest, and is worsened by repetitive muscle contractions. In-office diagnosis is based on these characteristics.

The edrophonium (Tensilon) test is the most important study used in the diagnosis of myasthenia gravis.[16] Tensilon inhibits anticholinesterase, the enzyme that breaks down acetylcholine at the neuromuscular junction. This increases the amount of acetylcholine available to react with the receptor sites, temporarily alleviating the muscle weakness. Thirty seconds after the intravenous administration of Tensilon, myasthenics will experience a brief resolution of their muscle weakness. Ptosis, motility deficits, and orbicularis weakness improve, which can be readily observed by the examiner. Because Tensilon can cause bradycardia, hypotension, or cardiac arrest, atropine should be made available during the test and is sometimes used prophylactically. Although these reactions

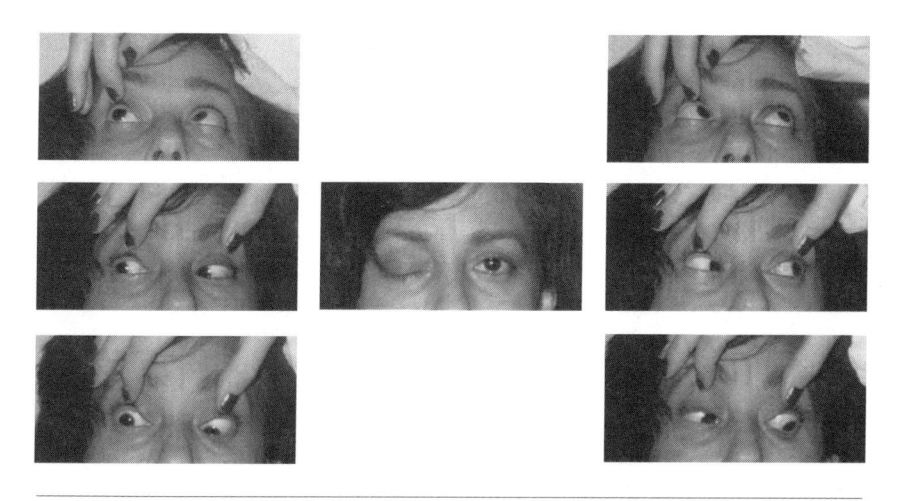

Figure 1.24 Ptosis and motility deficit mimicking third nerve palsy in a patient with myasthenia gravis.

are rare, resuscitation equipment should also be available. Patients with known cardiac disease are tested with caution and sometimes require electrocardiographic monitoring.

The rare occurrence of the aforementioned side effects limits testing with Tensilon to specialists in the appropriate medical setting. The optometrist faced with a suspicion of myasthenia must rely on some less known but extremely useful alternatives to the Tensilon test. These diagnostic tests are safe, in-office procedures that can provide strong evidence for the disorder before referral for confirmation with Tensilon or other neurologic testing.

The Sleep Test

The sleep test is a safe, in-office alternative to the Tensilon test.[17] It is based on the myasthenic characteristic of improvement after rest or sleep. It correlates well with the Tensilon test and is of great value in patients who are poor candidates for the Tensilon test. The following steps describe the procedure for conducting the sleep test:

1. The patient is photographed and ocular motility is measured as a baseline.

2. The patient is left in a dark room and is instructed to sleep or rest for 30 minutes.
3. Photographs and motility measurements are repeated and compared. Improvement of ptosis and ocular motility are suggestive of myasthenia gravis.

The sleep test is the most useful in-office test for the optometrist in diagnosing myasthenia with motility disturbances. Because most myasthenics will exhibit both ptosis and lid involvement and many will demonstrate orbicularis weakness, levator and orbicularis strength should always be evaluated in the patient suspected of having myasthenia gravis. Although electromyographic studies will demonstrate muscle weakness in ocular or general musculature, there are a number of simple ways to test for weakness of these two muscles.

Levator Function and Ptosis

Myasthenics often show marked improvement in ptosis after the application of ice to the eyelid. Cold temperature inhibits acetylcholinesterase (AChE), giving AChE a longer time to react with the reduced number of available receptor sites.[18] This improves neuromuscular transmission, resulting in a temporary resolution in muscle weakness. The test cannot be used to test for EOM weakness because the cold temperature does not penetrate deep enough. During testing, an ice pack is applied to a ptotic eyelid for 2 minutes, and the lid position is photographed or measured before and after application of the ice.

The testing of lid fatigue on sustained upgaze focuses on the fatigability of myasthenic muscles. The patient fixates a penlight in upgaze with instructions to refrain from blinking. One drop of topical anesthetic instilled into each eye helps eliminate the blink reflex. The suspect eyelid is observed for an increase in ptosis. If the examiner's arm tires before a noticeable lid droop occurs or worsens, the test is negative.

Cogan observed the lid twitch in one-half of his patients with ocular myasthenic signs.[19] He attributed it to fatigability with rapid recovery of myasthenic muscles. The patient's gaze is directed downward for 10–20 seconds. The patient is then instructed to make a vertical saccade back to primary position by holding an appropriate fixation target. The

Figure 1.25
Orbicularis strength can be tested by instructing the patient to squeeze the eyes shut while the examiner attempts to open them.

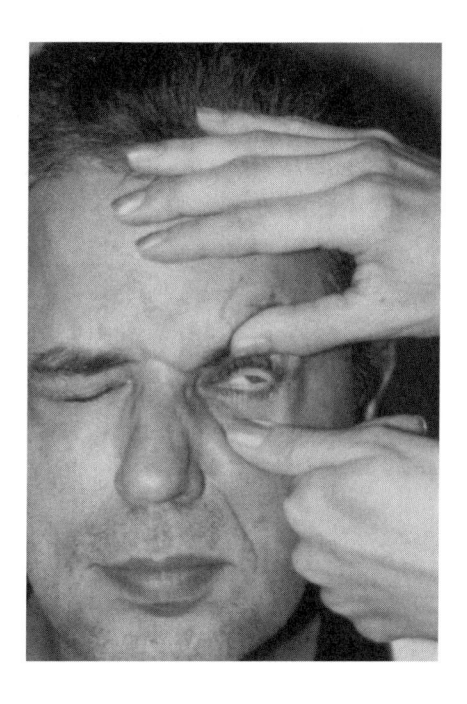

examiner should watch for an upward twitch of the eyelid when the eye returns to primary fixation.

Orbicularis Weakness

Orbicularis strength is evaluated by forced lid closure. The patient is instructed to close the eyelids tightly "as if there were soap in them." The examiner grasps the upper and lower lids with both thumbs as he or she attempts to manually open the eyes (Figure 1.25). Normally, this is difficult to overcome without everting the eyelid (a fact that often becomes apparent when attempting to instill drops into the eyes of a child). Eyelids that can be easily pried apart suggest orbicularis weakness.

Another sign of orbicularis weakness is incomplete eyelid closure. The patient is instructed to gently close his or her eyes as if sleeping. With a penlight, the examiner checks to see if the eyes are completely closed or if scleral tissue is visible through partially opened eyelids.

Billing and Reimbursement

Many of the tests in this chapter fall under the procedure of sensorimotor examination, which is defined as measuring ocular deviation in numerous positions of gaze. The Current Procedural Terminology (CPT) code for this is 92060, and reimbursement is approximately $40, although fees vary by carrier. Other tests in this chapter do not have a specific code but may support increasing the office visit code to a higher level.

Related International Classification of Diseases-9 (ICD-9) Terminology

Third nerve palsy (partial)	378.51
Third nerve palsy (total)	378.52
Fourth nerve palsy	378.53
Sixth nerve palsy	378.54
INO	378.86
Supranuclear paralysis (e.g., skew deviation)	356.8
Myasthenia gravis	358.0
Graves' disease	242.0
Paralytic strabismus (unspecified)	378.0
Diplopia	368.2

References

1. Burian HM, von Noorden GK. Binocular Vision and Ocular Motility: Theory and Management of Strabismus. St. Louis: Mosby, 1974;189–191, 260–261.
2. Critchley M. Types of visual perseveration; "palinopsia" and "illusionary visual spread." Brain 1951;74:265–299.
3. Safran AB, Kline LB, Glaser JS, et al. Television-induced formed visual hallucinations and cerebral diplopia. Br J Ophthalmol 1981;65:707–711.
4. Lancaster WB. Detecting, measuring, plotting and interpreting ocular deviations. Arch Opthalmol 1939;22:867–882.

5. Parks MM. Isolated cyclovertical muscle palsy. Arch Ophthalmol 1958;60:1027.
6. Bielschowsky A. Lectures on Motor Anomalies. Hanover, NH: Dartmouth College Publications, 1943;74–79.
7. Metz JS, Scott AB, O'Meara D, Stewart HL. Ocular saccades in lateral rectus palsy. Arch Ophthalmol 1970;84:453–457.
8. Gorman CA. Temporal relationship between onset of Graves' ophthalmopathy and diagnosis of thyrotoxicosis. Mayo Clin Proc 1983;58:515.
9. Zappia RJ, Winkelman JZ, Gay AJ. Intraocular pressure changes in normal subjects and the adhesive muscle syndrome. Am J Ophthalmol 1971;71:880–883.
10. Feldon SE, Levin L. Graves' ophthalmopathy: V. Aetology of upper eyelid retraction in Graves' ophthalmopathy. Br J Ophthalmol 1990;74:484–485.
11. Grove AS Jr. Upper eyelid retraction and Graves' disease. Ophthalmol 1981;88:499–506.
12. Werner SC, Ingbar SH. The Thyroid: A Fundamental and Clinical Text (3rd ed). New York: Harper & Row, 1971;536.
13. Keane JR. Ocular skew deviation: analysis of 100 cases. Arch Neurol 1975;32:185–190.
14. Drachman DB, Adams RN, Stanley EF, Pestronk A. Mechanisms of acetylcholine receptor loss in myasthenia gravis. J Neurol Neurosurg Psychiatr 1980;43:601–610.
15. Evoli A, Tonali P, Bartoccione E, Lo Monaco M. Ocular myasthenia: diagnostic and therapeutic problems. Acta Neurol Scand 1988;77:31–35.
16. Osserman KE, Kaplan LI. Rapid diagnostic test for myasthenia gravis—increased muscle strength, without fasciculations, after intravenous administration of edrophonium (Tensilon) chloride. JAMA 1952;105:265–268.
17. Odel J, Winterkorn J, Behrens M. The sleep test for myasthenia gravis—a safe alternative to Tensilon. J Clin Neuro-ophthalmol 1991;11:288–292.
18. Sethi KD, Rivner MH, Swift TR. Ice-pack test in myasthenia gravis. Ann NY Acad Sci 1987;505:584–587.
19. Cogan DG. Myasthenia gravis: a review of the disease and a description of lid twitch as a characteristic sign. Arch Ophthalmol 1965;74:217.

2

Pupil Evaluation

Pupillary function is controlled both by the sympathetic and parasympathetic limbs of the autonomic nervous system. Signs that something is awry in one of these two systems include pupils that are of unequal size, that are of irregular shape, or that are poorly responsive to light and accommodation. Such disturbances in pupil size or function can be indicative of anterior visual pathway or other nervous system disease. Often, the optometrist is the first member of the health care team to recognize the abnormality and as such, should be familiar with the diagnosis, workup, and management. Not only is it crucial to recognize a condition that has potentially serious implications, but it is also important to realize the benignity of certain pupillary disturbances to avoid what can often be expensive and unproductive medical evaluations.

Parasympathetic Control and the Pupillary Light Reflex

Afferent pupillomotor input begins with stimulation of retinal photoreceptor cells that transfer information to ganglion cells. The information is carried intracranially via the optic nerve and optic tracts, with a hemidecussation of axons at the chiasm (Figure 2.1). Pupillomotor fibers bypass the lateral geniculate nucleus and travel to the pretectal nuclei in the mesencephalon via the brachium of the superior colliculus. Fibers then synapse in the visceral nuclei of the oculomotor complex after decussating both dorsally and ventrally around the sylvian aqueduct. Efferent axons arise from the oculomotor complex and

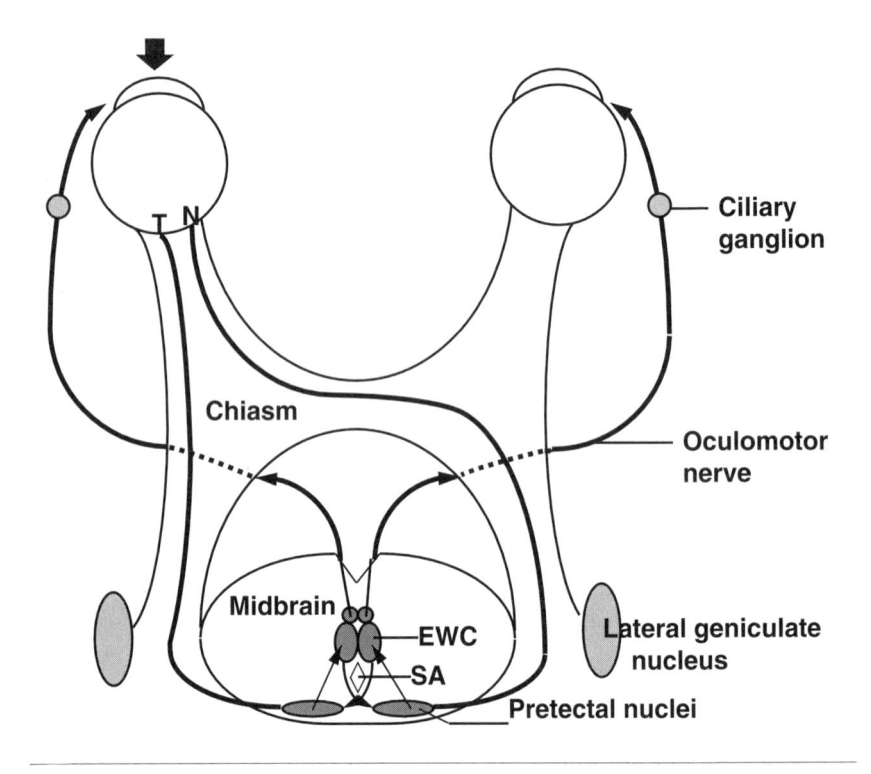

Figure 2.1 The chiasm and rostral midbrain showing the afferent and efferent pupillomotor pathway. Pupillomotor fibers from the nasal retina (N) cross in the chiasm while temporal fibers (T) do not. (EWC = Edinger-Westphal complex; SA = sylvian aqueduct.) (Reprinted with permission from P Modica. Afferent pupillary defects and the swinging flashlight test. What you thought you already knew. Optom Clin 1996;5:1–15.)

travel rostrally with the third nerve fascicles and nerve. They enter the orbit in the inferior division of the third cranial nerve and then synapse in the ciliary ganglion. From there they travel to the iris sphincter via the short ciliary nerves to control pupillary constriction. Activation of this reflex arc begins with light stimulation to the eye and results in pupil constriction. Because of multiple decussations of this pathway, unilateral stimulation results in equal pupillary constriction in both eyes.

The Near Reflex

The triad of pupillary miosis, convergence, and accommodation is known as the *near reflex*. This triad is also under parasympathetic control and occurs when fixation is shifted from a distance to a near target. Although the light reflex and the near reflex have separate afferent pathways, both have a common efferent pathway in the third nerve fascicles that synapses in the ciliary ganglion.

Sympathetic Control

Pupil dilation is controlled by the sympathetic limb of the autonomic nervous system, which originates in the hypothalamus. The sympathetic pathway is composed of a three-neuron arc. The first-order (central) neuron descends from the posterolateral area of the hypothalamus through the mesencephalon, pons, and medulla and synapses in the intermediolateral gray substance of the cervical or thoracic spinal cord (C8 or T1). From there, axons of the second-order (intermediate or preganglionic) neuron exit the spinal cord via the ventral spinal roots and enter the paravertebral sympathetic chain via the white rami communicantes. At this point, the axons are closely associated with the apex of the lung and may be affected by pulmonary lesions. The fibers then ascend to the superior cervical ganglion located at the base of the skull, where they synapse. The third-order (postganglionic) neuron arises from the superior cervical ganglion and travels rostrally with the common carotid artery. At the bifurcation of the internal and external carotid arteries, oculosympathetic fibers ascend in the internal carotid artery, while those fibers destined to control sweating of the face will travel with the external carotid artery. Oculosympathetic fibers travel with the internal carotid artery to the cavernous sinus, where they briefly join the sixth cranial nerve. Finally, they join the ophthalmic division of the trigeminal nerve to enter the orbit. Fibers reach the iris dilator muscle via the long posterior ciliary nerves. The sympathetic pupillary pathway is summarized in Figure 2.2.

The first two neurons make up the preganglionic portion of the three-neuron pathway, whereas the postganglionic portion consists of the

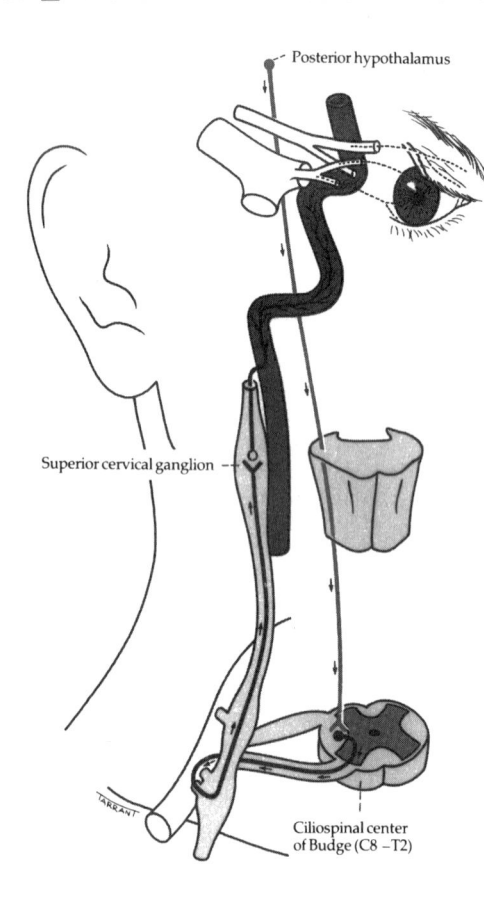

Figure 2.2
Summary of the oculosympathetic pathway. (Reprinted with permission from JJ Kanski. Clinical Ophthalmology [2nd ed]. Oxford: Butterworth–Heinemann, 1989; 475.)

Labels: Posterior hypothalamus; Superior cervical ganglion; Ciliospinal center of Budge (C8–T2)

third-order neuron. Disruptions along any part of this three-neuron pathway result in oculosympathetic paresis.

History Taking

Patients presenting for evaluation of disturbances of pupillary function include the following:

1. Patients with anisocoria
2. Patients with impaired pupillary responses
3. Patients with irregularities in pupil shape

Generally speaking, patients with abnormal pupillary function present with minimal symptomatology. Symptoms may include cosmetic complaints related to differences in pupil sizes; photophobia (in patients with abnormally dilated pupils); accommodative dysfunction (in patients with tonic pupils); diplopia, ptosis, and perhaps pain (in patients with third nerve palsy); ptosis alone (in patients with Horner's syndrome); and vision loss (in patients with optic nerve disease and afferent pupillary defects [APDs]). In most cases, abnormalities are not brought to the attention of the clinician by the patient, but rather are noted on routine examination or by referral from another physician.

History taking of the patient with anisocoria should begin with questioning the patient as to awareness of the condition. If the patient is aware of the abnormality, noting its onset is not only helpful in sorting out its cause, but also in determining its management. For example, a recent onset of a Horner's syndrome in an adult is more likely to represent a lung malignancy requiring a medical workup than a long-standing and well-documented Horner's syndrome. Just like history taking in diplopic patients, medical history plays an important role in patients with pupillary abnormalities. Both the general health and past health history should be questioned in detail because they may provide valuable clues with regard to etiology of the patient's condition. Furthermore, patients should be questioned with regard to household medications, occupation, and recent activities to rule out accidental instillation of mydriatic agents. Table 2.1 summarizes some important aspects of the patient history and possible related pupillary abnormalities.

Materials Required for Evaluation of Pupillary Function

A complete evaluation of pupillary function does not require complicated equipment. Most of the essential materials are familiar to the optometrist and are easily obtained.

1. Appropriate light source should be capable of providing a range of illuminations from dim to bright (a handheld transilluminator or binocular indirect ophthalmoscope are ideal).
2. Pupil gauges are available in 1-mm increments.

Table 2.1 Patient History and Potentially Related Pupil Abnormalities

History	Considerations
Syphilis	Argyll-Robertson pupils; neuropathic tonic pupils
Blurred vision	Tonic pupil; pharmacologic pupil; afferent pupillary defect
Diplopia	Third nerve palsy; dorsal midbrain syndrome
Arm pain/smoking	Horner's syndrome
Ocular trauma	Local tonic pupil; afferent pupillary defect
Head trauma	Third nerve palsy; dorsal midbrain syndrome; afferent pupillary defect; Horner's syndrome
Medication	Pharmacologic pupil
Hypertension	Aneurysmal third nerve palsy; afferent pupillary defect
Thoracic or cervical surgery/injury	Horner's syndrome
Diabetes	Tonic pupil; optic nerve or retinal disease with afferent pupillary defect

3. Topical, diagnostic pharmaceutical agents include diluted pilocarpine and phenylephrine solutions, 1% hydroxyamphetamine solution, and 6–10% cocaine solution. The latter two are limited in availability: cocaine, due to its classification as a controlled substance, and hydroxyamphetamine, due to manufacturer limitations.

4. Slit-lamp biomicroscope examination is essential to rule out structural abnormalities of the iris, which may impair pupillary responses.

5. Neutral-density filters that range from 0.3 to 1.2 log units are used in the grading of APDs.

Performing the Test: Six Important Steps

Ruling Out/Assessing Anisocoria

Before beginning any evaluation of the pupil, it is first necessary to measure pupil sizes in both bright and dim illumination. This is important for two reasons: It identifies an anisocoria, which could confound the results of the swinging flashlight test, and in the patient with anisocoria, it identifies the limb of the autonomic nervous system that is at fault.

Figure 2.3
Pupillary measurements in bright illumination. Pupil gauges are readily available from a number of manufacturers. (Reprinted with permission from P Modica. Afferent pupillary defects and the swinging flashlight test. What you thought you already knew. Optom Clin 1996;5:1–15.)

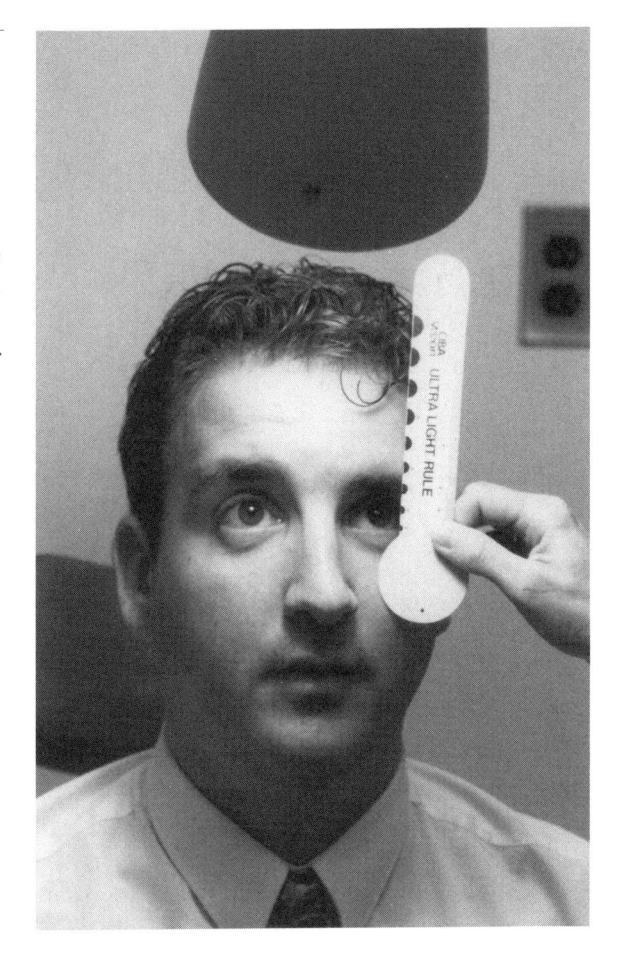

Measurement in bright illumination is best accomplished by having room illumination at its brightest and a gooseneck lamp directed toward the patient's eyes. Patients should fixate a distant target to maximize sphincter relaxation and to avoid a confounding near response. A pupil gauge held adjacent to each pupil obtains the most accurate measurement (Figure 2.3). To measure the pupils in dim illumination, all lights should be turned off to promote a widely dilated pupil. A penlight or transilluminator is held below the chin and directed upward (Figure 2.4). The light should be as dim as possible, yet provide just enough illumination to visualize the pupil margins.

Anisocoria that is more pronounced in dim illumination suggests sympathetic paralysis in the eye with the smaller pupil as seen in

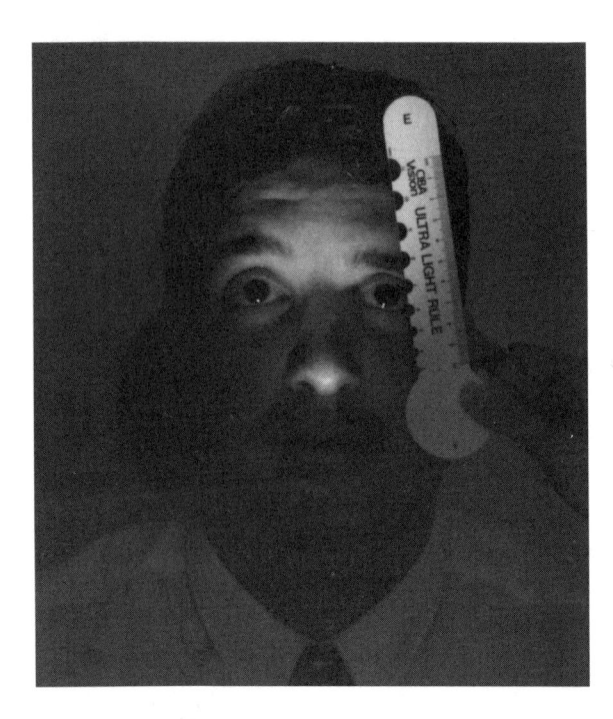

Figure 2.4
Pupillary measurements in dim illumination. A penlight or transilluminator enables visualization of pupils in a darkened room. (Reprinted with permission from P Modica. Afferent pupillary defects and the swinging flashlight test. What you thought you already knew. Optom Clin 1996;5:1–15.)

Horner's syndrome. Anisocoria that is more pronounced in bright illumination suggests an impaired efferent limb of the parasympathetic system in the eye with the larger pupil (Figure 2.5). Benign, physiologic anisocoria is characterized by anisocoria that remains the same in both bright and dim illumination and normal pupillary responses.

■ The Direct and Consensual Response

An intact pupillary response to light depends on an intact afferent and efferent pupillary pathway. When the direct light response is impaired, further information is gained by assessing the integrity of the consensual response. The direct light response is assessed by darkening the room to maximize pupil dilation. Fixation is directed at a distant target near the ceiling to eliminate accommodation and raise the pupillary axis so that the light source does not obstruct it. An appropriate light source is important. A general rule of thumb is that older patients with more sluggish pupil responses require more intense stimuli, such as a binocular indirect

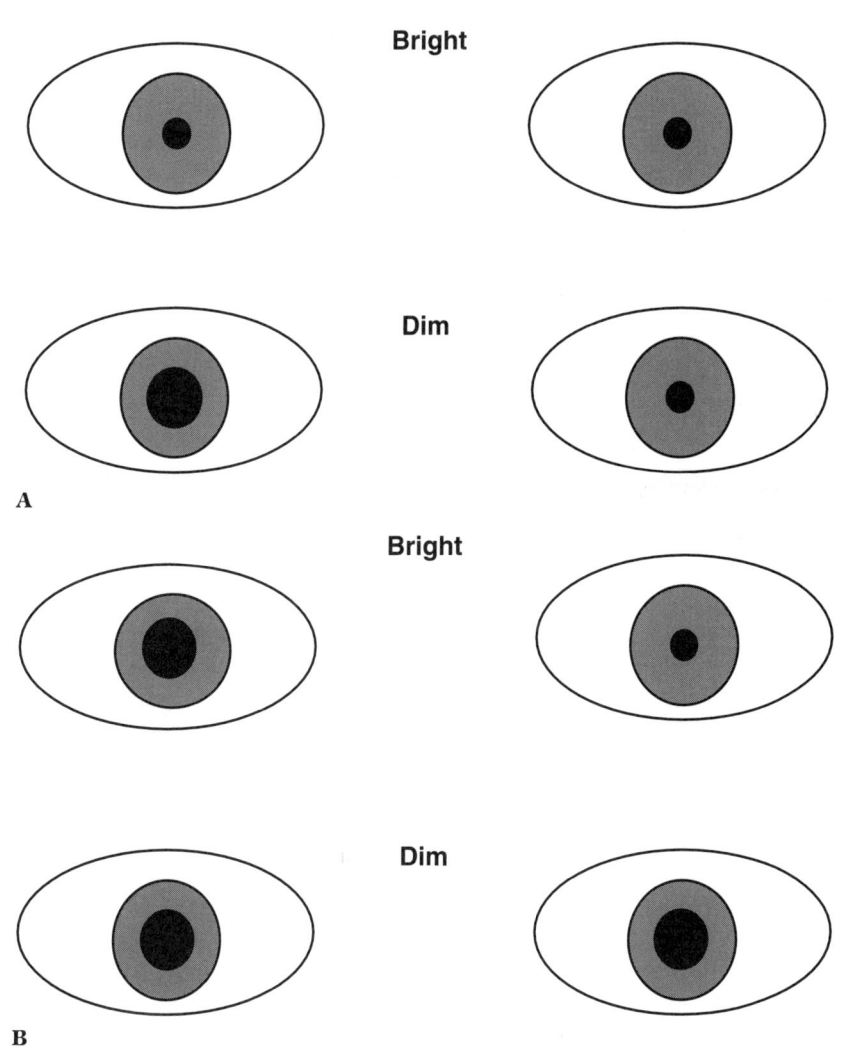

Figure 2.5 (A) Anisocoria that is more pronounced in dim illumination indicates sympathetic paralysis in the eye with the smaller pupil.
(B) Anisocoria that is more pronounced in bright illumination indicates parasympathetic paralysis in the eye with the larger pupil.

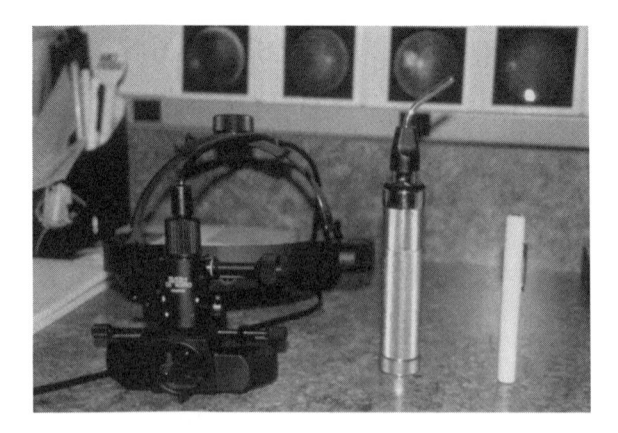

Figure 2.6
Appropriate light sources for pupil testing. The ideal stimulus is determined by the individual responses of the patient.

ophthalmoscope, whereas younger patients with brisk responses can be tested with penlights (Figure 2.6). The light source is held approximately 1 inch from the eye so that the fellow eye is not affected by stray light, and it is directed into the eyes from slightly below the pupillary axis to avoid the effects of accommodation. The stimulus is presented for approximately 3 seconds. The normal pupillary response to light consists of a brisk constriction followed by a slight redilation due to physiologic play in the iris sphincter and retinal adaptation. This response is dependent on both an intact afferent and efferent pupillary pathway. Observing the consensual response of the fellow eye is helpful in diagnosing afferent pathway disease and is accomplished with the swinging flashlight test.[1]

The swinging flashlight test begins by presenting the stimulus for a fast count of three and then moving the light as quickly as possible across the bridge of the nose to the fellow eye for a fast count of three. Moving the light quickly minimizes redilation, allowing better comparison between the two eyes. When the light first enters the fellow eye, there will typically be a slight constriction followed by a slight redilation. The light is swung back and forth so that each eye is stimulated for a total of three times. The examiner observes the speed and extent of the initial constriction as well as any redilation and compares the two eyes.

In a normal individual, the direct response should equal the consensual response seen in the fellow eye. In afferent system disease, the direct response is diminished or absent. When a reduced afferent signal reaches the pretectal nuclei, a reduced efferent signal is generated, resulting in a reduced pupillary constriction to light in both eyes. When the light is moved from the impaired eye to the normal eye, a better afferent signal results in a better efferent response and, hence, better constriction in both eyes. Therefore,

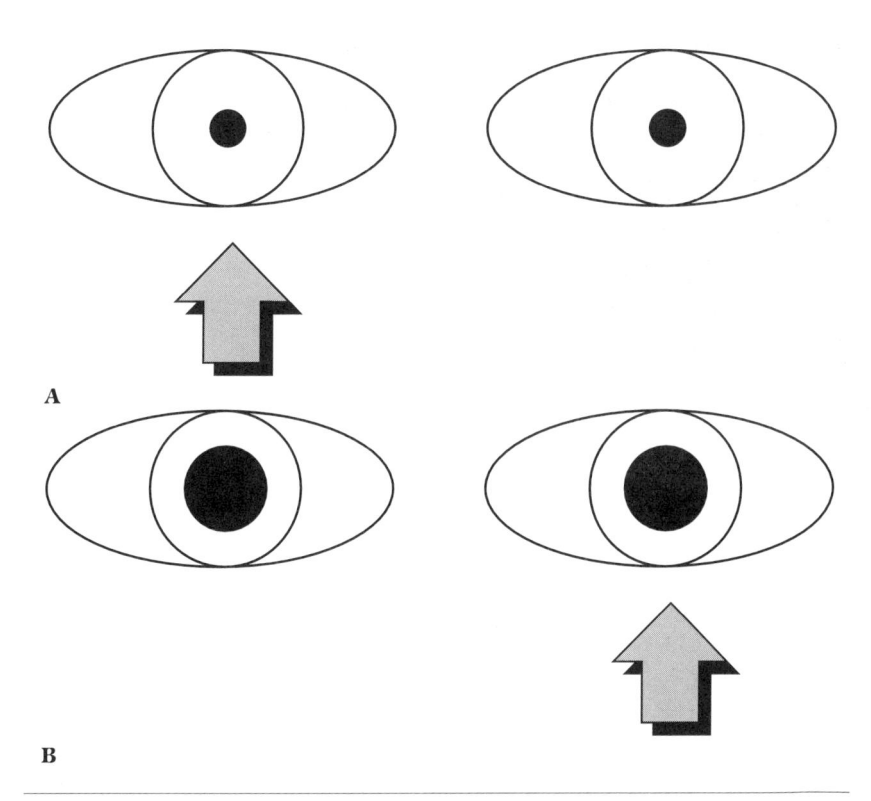

Figure 2.7 Schematic diagram of pupillary findings in a patient with a left afferent pupillary defect. (A) When the right eye is stimulated, both pupils constrict. (B) When the left eye is stimulated, both pupils dilate. (Reprinted with permission from P Modica. Afferent pupillary defects and the swinging flashlight test. What you thought you already knew. Optom Clin 1996;5:1–15.)

patients with APDs will show bilateral constriction of the pupils when the normal eye is stimulated and bilateral dilation when the defective eye is stimulated (Figure 2.7). Because only the stimulated eye is observed, the examiner will note constriction in the "good eye" and dilation in the "bad eye" as the light is alternated. In an eye that has a diminished light response from efferent system disease, there will be no direct light response, but because an intact efferent signal reaches the pretectal nuclei, the consensual response of the fellow eye will be normal. Likewise, when the light is moved to the fellow eye, it will maintain this constriction (although some fluctuations will be noted due to physiologic unrest).

The Near Response and Pupillary Light–Near Dissociation

The near response is assessed by instructing the patient to fixate a near target. The target should be interesting enough to provoke an adequate accommodative response. Often, the effort to accommodate is inadequate and can mislead the observer. For this reason, the near response is only important when it is observed to be better than the light response, a phenomenon known as *pupillary light–near dissociation*. Pupillary light–near dissociation is an important finding in a number of pupillary disturbances. In cases in which poor vision prevents fixation on a near target, the patient's own finger held at close range provides an adequate near stimulus (Figure 2.8). Even if the target cannot be visualized, proprioceptive input guides the patient. Patients can also be asked to cross their eyes voluntarily to elicit a near response.[2] If convergence is not noted when testing the near response, the patient is unable or is not making an effort to accommodate.

Although the near reflex and light reflex have different afferent input to the third nerve nuclear complex, they both share common efferent pathways via the third nerve fascicles. If there is a disturbance in the afferent light reflex pathway from the photoreceptors to the pretectal nuclei, the near reflex will remain intact. If there is an efferent disorder such as is seen in a third nerve palsy involving the pupil, there will be a diminished pupillary response to both light and near.

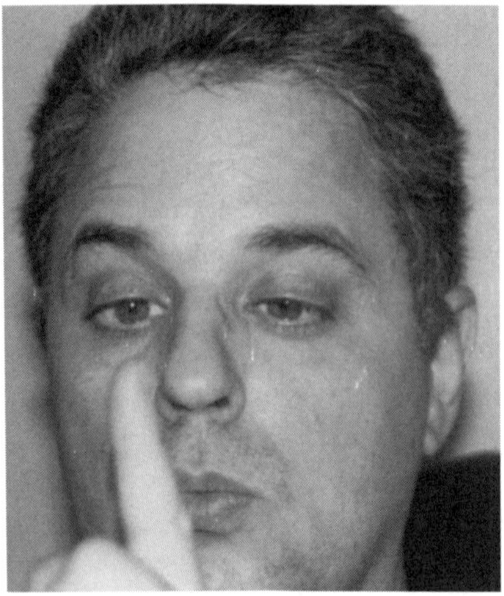

Figure 2.8
The near response can be evaluated by having the patient fixate his or her own finger held at close range.

■ Observing the Eyelid

The eyelid and pupil share an important relationship, and a careful inspection of the eyelid position is an important part of a complete pupillary examination. The examiner should pay close attention to eyelid position in the eye with abnormal pupil responses to rule out ptosis or eyelid retraction.

Ptosis with an abnormally small pupil is indicative of Horner's syndrome; ptosis and an abnormally large pupil may be seen in third nerve palsy or from blunt trauma that damages both the pupil and eyelid musculature. Bilateral eyelid retraction with mid-dilated, light-near dissociated pupils may be due to bilateral interruption of afferent signals from rostral midbrain disease.

■ Biomicroscopic Evaluation

Biomicroscopy allows the examiner to rule out or diagnose local abnormalities to the iris and pupillary margin that have the potential to impair the light response, near response, or both. Such abnormalities include posterior synechiae, sphincter tears, and other signs of trauma or surgery, as well as irregularities associated with impaired innervation. The light source on the biomicroscope can be used to detect areas of subtle pupillary reaction that are not easily detected with a penlight.

Impaired pupil responses from blunt trauma may be due to efferent impairment from structural disease or concomitant optic neuropathy with afferent impairment. Tonic pupils are classically associated with sectorial responses to light with irregular pupillary margins.

■ Pharmacologic Testing

The use of topical pharmaceutical agents is necessary in certain pupillary disorders to confirm the diagnosis or to localize the disturbance in the affected pathway. It plays an important role in the diagnosis and localization of Horner's syndrome, in the diagnosis of postganglionic denervation of the sympathetic and parasympathetic pupillary disturbances, and in the confirmation of accidental pharmacologic pupillary dilation. Pharmacologic testing and its interpretation are further discussed with each disorder.

Abnormal Pupil Types

The optometrist should be familiar with six types of abnormal pupils:

1. The APD
2. The tonic pupil
3. The pupil in midbrain disease
4. Horner's syndrome
5. The pupil in third nerve palsy
6. The pharmacologically dilated pupil

■ Afferent Pupillary Defect

Disease affecting the afferent pupillomotor pathway from the retinal ganglion cells to the pretectal nuclei can result in an APD. The swinging flashlight test originally described by Levatin[1] is the key diagnostic test that reveals constriction to a light stimulus in a normal eye and dilation or "escape" in the eye with a defective afferent pathway when the eyes are alternately stimulated. Pupillary studies have shown that patients with APDs will also have an initial constriction that is slower and/or reduced in amplitude relative to the normal eye.[3] With this in mind, the examiner should not only look for pupillary escape, but should also observe the speed and extent of the brief initial constriction in both eyes.

Sources of Error in the Swinging Flashlight Test

Stimulus Intensity The ideal light intensity and source necessary for proper pupil testing is controversial,[4-6] and there is no uniformly accepted stimulus to perform the test. Stimulus intensity is gauged on an individual basis and should be dictated by the response of the pupil.[7] A light source that is too dim will generate a pupillary response that is too sluggish and of diminished magnitude to allow optimal observation of a subtle APD.[4] A light source that is too bright will result in a pupillary spasm[8] and cause a bright afterimage,[9] resulting in a prolonged initial constriction and a masking of the redilation phase. The examiner should begin with a penlight or transilluminator with fresh batteries, and if the direct response is not sufficient, should switch to a more intense stimulus such as the binocular indirect ophthalmoscope set at six volts.

Test Speed As previously mentioned, the direct light response in a normal patient consists of an initial constriction to light followed by a slight dilation. The examiner should allow enough time for the complete cycle to occur before switching the light to the other eye. Although a fast count of three is the recommended guideline, speed of pupillary responses varies from patient to patient. Therefore, test speed should vary accordingly. For brisk responses, the count should be faster, and the count should be slower for more sluggish responses. A more important consideration is the rhythm of the test. Light that is held on one eye longer than the other may result in a false APD in the eye with the longer stimulus duration due to unequal bleaching of retinal photoreceptors. This is an important consideration, as the examiner will often overstimulate a suspect eye in an effort to detect the APD.

Physiologic Hippus or Pupillary Unrest It is often difficult to distinguish physiologic hippus and pupillary unrest from the pupillary escape seen in optic nerve disease. It is traditionally recommended that in patients with active pupillary unrest, the amount of redilation should be compared in each eye. An eye that consistently has a greater redilation has an APD.[1,9] This comparison is often a difficult one because such differences in pupillary movement are subtle and cannot be compared objectively without the use of pupillography equipment available to researchers. Furthermore, Cox[10] has shown that the pupillary escape of optic nerve disease described by Levatin[11] is a less reliable indicator of an APD and that it is often more helpful to eliminate this often confounding aspect of the test by observing only the magnitude and speed of the initial constriction. This is accomplished by increasing the speed of the test. The examiner watches the speed and extent of the initial constriction and then switches the light to the fellow eye before the redilation phase occurs. The result is that the speed of the swinging flashlight test increases substantially. If the initial constriction is absent or slowed relative to the fellow eye, an APD may be diagnosed.

Physiologic Anisocoria The presence of anisocoria is an important source of error in the swinging flashlight test and one that frequently results in unnecessary referrals to specialists or unnecessary additional testing. Anisocoria can cause a pseudo-APD in the eye with the larger pupil; the examiner will often misinterpret the larger pupil size as a redilation. This can be avoided by checking the pupils for anisocoria in both bright and dim illumination before checking for an APD.

Paying close attention to potential sources of error is particularly important in ensuring detection of mild APDs. Even when conditions are optimal, the APD is often too subtle to allow easy detection. Varying the stimulus intensity, test speed, or both as described is often helpful. In most cases, an equivocal APD can be made more obvious by placing a 0.3 log neutral-density filter before the suspect eye while observing the pupils during the swinging flashlight test[9] (Figure 2.9). The filter "magnifies" the APD to a more easily detectable intensity, thereby confirming its presence. On the other hand, a 0.3 log filter placed over the normal eye will have little effect because it has the net effect of canceling out the APD in the suspect eye.

Indirect Afferent Pupillary Defect Too often, examiners fail to perform the swinging flashlight test in patients with a unilaterally fixed pupil because they think that both pupils need to be working to perform the test. It is necessary to have only one normally reactive iris sphincter to determine the presence of an APD in either eye. When a fixed pupil is present, as may occur postsurgically, pharmacologically, after trauma, or from posterior synechia, only the pupil with the working iris sphincter is observed while performing the swinging flashlight test. The pupillary findings are interpreted as follows. If an APD exists in the eye with the reactive pupil, then that pupil will constrict more with consensual stimulation than with direct stimulation (Figure 2.10). If the defect exists in the eye with the fixed pupil, the reactive pupil will constrict more with direct stimulation than consensual stimulation (Figure 2.11).

Grading Afferent Pupillary Defects

A complete pupillary assessment should include comments regarding the magnitude of the APD. The conventional method of grading APDs consists of the examiner assigning a grade of 1+ to 4+ based on the apparent magnitude of the APD. Unfortunately, grading this way is arbitrary and often inaccurate. For example, a young patient with brisk pupils has an easily recognizable APD whereas in an elderly patient with more slowly responsive pupils, an APD of the same magnitude is not quite so obvious.

Figure 2.9
(A) Neutral-density filters are inexpensive and can be purchased at photographic supply stores. (B) Placement of a neutral-density filter while performing the swinging flashlight test. Note that the pupils are easily observed through the filter. (Reprinted with permission from P Modica. Afferent pupillary defects and the swinging flashlight test. What you thought you already knew. Optom Clin 1996;5:1–15.)

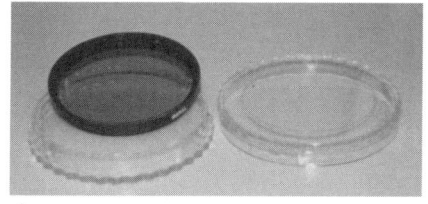

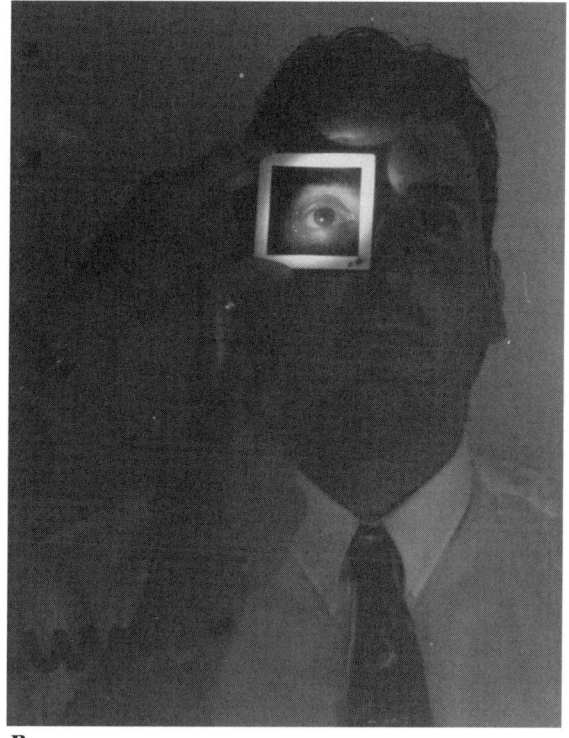

For this reason, the examiner will often overestimate a mild APD in a young patient and underestimate a less obvious but higher magnitude APD in an elderly patient.

An objective method of grading APDs is with the use of neutral-density filters.[9] A series of four neutral-density filters, ranging from 0.3 log units to 1.2 log units in increments of 0.3 log units, can be purchased inexpensively from a photography store. If an APD exists, filters are placed in front of the normal eye, gradually increasing the density in

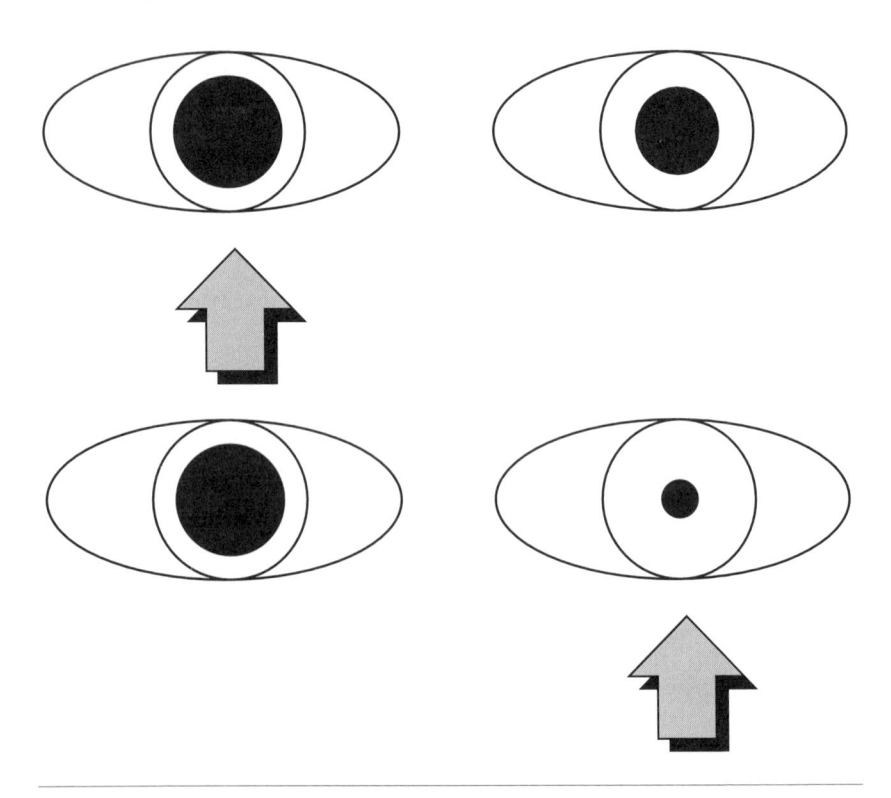

Figure 2.10 An indirect afferent pupillary defect in a fixed, dilated right pupil. When the right eye is stimulated, the left pupil dilates. When the left pupil is stimulated, it constricts. (Reprinted with permission from P Modica. Afferent pupillary defects and the swinging flashlight test. What you thought you already knew. Optom Clin 1996; 5:1–15.)

0.3 log increments, cutting the amount of light entering the eye until the APD can no longer be seen. This is the point at which the density of the defect is balanced with the neutral-density filter. Additional filters should then overshoot the balance point, causing a reversal of the APD. The APD can now be graded by simply assigning the density of the filter(s) used to neutralize the defect. For example, if the defect is balanced with a 0.9 log filter, it is recorded as a 0.9 log APD. The filters are additive so that a set of four filters can be used in combination to measure defects of up to 3.0 log units, and additional filters can be pur-

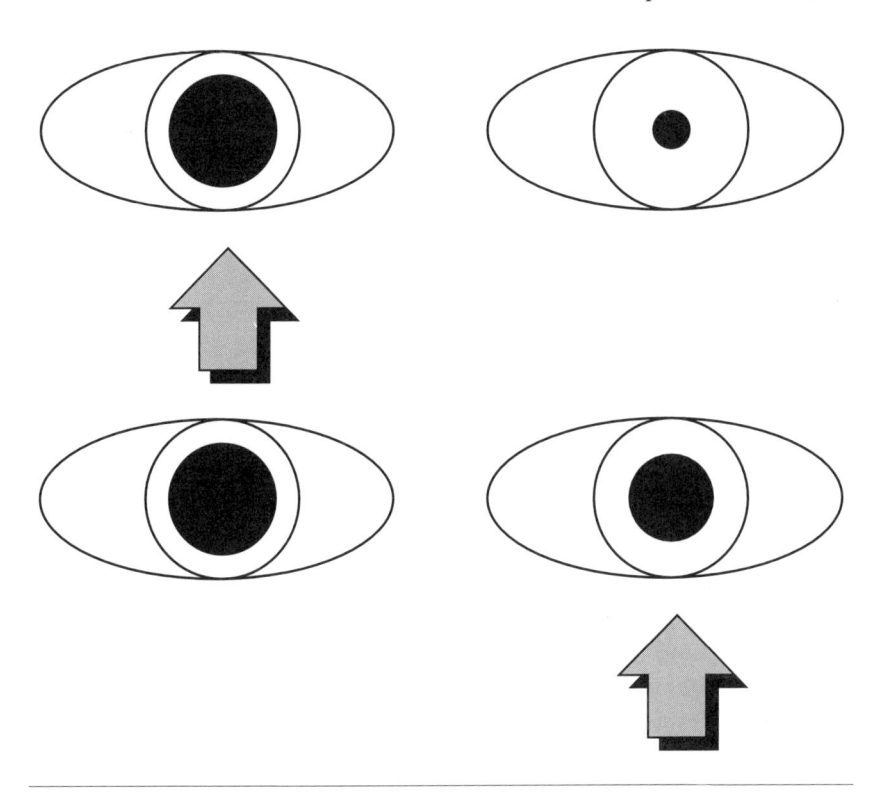

Figure 2.11 An indirect afferent pupillary defect in the left eye of a patient with a fixed, dilated right pupil. When the right eye is stimulated, the left pupil constricts. When the left eye is stimulated, it dilates. (Reprinted with permission from P Modica. Afferent pupillary defects and the swinging flashlight test. What you thought you already knew. Optom Clin 1996;5:1–15.)

chased if the examiner needs to go higher. Beyond 3.6 log units, grading loses its accuracy.

Filters alone or in a combination exceeding 1.2 log units will be too dim to observe the pupil while looking through them, and the examiner must peek around the filter to observe the pupil. When using neutral-density filters, the examiner must work quickly because unilateral placement of the filters results in asymmetric bleaching of the retinal photoreceptors. When this occurs, more and more filters will be needed to balance the defect, and the measurements will be overestimated. Therefore, an attempt should be made to balance the defect with as few swings as possible. If more than three swings are needed, the filter should be taken away, and both eyes should be flashed with the light to balance the retinal bleach before continuing.[9]

Although the use of neutral-density filters is the preferred method of grading APDs, they may not be practical for everyone. A grading system has been proposed that is based on the characteristics of the pupillary responses during the swinging flashlight test.[11] The swinging flashlight test is performed, using a stimulus time of 3 seconds per eye. The APD is graded initially on a scale of I–III based on the following criteria:

> Grade I—There is a weak initial constriction to the stimulus, with a greater redilation relative to the fellow eye.
> Grade II—There is an initial stall before the pupil constricts, followed by a greater redilation relative to the fellow eye.
> Grade III—There is an immediate redilation to the stimulus. If the APD is determined to be either grade I or grade II, the results are recorded. If, however, there is an immediate redilation to the stimulus (grade III), further evaluation is needed to determine the magnitude of the APD. The normal eye is next stimulated for 6 seconds to bleach the photoreceptors and weaken its "pupil power." This has the effect of weakening the response of the good eye so that the suspect eye can now be compared with a weaker eye. The light is then swung back to the weak eye. If an initial constriction is observed, the APD remains a grade III.
> Grades IV and V are distinguished by the following characteristics:
> Grade IV—There is an immediate dilation followed by a constriction.
> Grade V—There is an immediate dilation with no secondary constriction.

By providing clear guidelines with respect to the observed behavior of the pupil, this scale puts some objectivity back into the grading of the defects. Although the extra step takes a little bit longer than the traditional swinging flashlight test, the actual grading is faster than with the use of filters. The authors who originally described the technique have shown it to correlate well with the use of filters, and it is not affected by intraobserver variability.[11] It is also consistent with grading scales derived from the use of neutral-density filters. One minor problem with this grading system is that it is very difficult to distinguish a grade I from a grade II APD.

As with any disease process, clinicians need to know whether a patient is stable or if there has been progression. Although grading the APD is one way of monitoring the disease, it should be understood that there are other clinical correlates that are important adjuncts to the swinging flashlight test. Color vision, Snellen acuity, contrast sensitivity, ophthalmoscopy, and threshold visual field testing are also important clinical correlates. Although they should be evaluated collectively, the threshold visual field is perhaps the most important tool if each were considered independently. APDs are associated with, and correlate very nicely with visual field defects.[12,13] A clear advantage to using threshold perimetry as a monitoring tool over simply measuring an APD by the described methods is that it is more sensitive to subtle changes in optic nerve function and therefore a better indicator of progression.

■ Tonic Pupils

Damage to the ciliary ganglion from trauma or disease results in postganglionic denervation of the efferent pupillomotor pathway with a tonic pupillary response. Tonic pupils are characterized by postganglionic denervation with supersensitivity to dilute pilocarpine solutions, light-near dissociation, sector paralysis with an absent or sectorial light response, and a sluggish near response with slow redilation. They can be categorized into three basic types[14]:

1. Local tonic pupils occur from orbital trauma or infection that damages the ciliary ganglion or short ciliary nerves.
2. Neuropathic tonic pupils occur in the setting of generalized peripheral or autonomic nervous system disease that also involves the ciliary ganglion or short ciliary nerves. They are often seen in syphilis, diabetes, and chronic alcoholism.
3. Adie's pupil, or idiopathic tonic pupil, occurs in healthy patients and in the absence of orbital trauma, surgery, infection, or nervous system disease. It is by far the most common of the tonic pupils; therefore, its diagnosis is emphasized here. In addition to the aforementioned characteristics of tonic pupil, most patients with Adie's tonic pupil have reduced or absent tendon reflexes despite an otherwise normal neurologic examination.

Characteristics of Adie's Tonic Pupil

Adie's tonic pupil occurs most commonly in women between 20 and 50 years of age.[14] Most patients are affected unilaterally; however, the fellow eye may be involved months to years later. Simultaneous involvement may also occur initially. Symptoms include blurred vision at near from accommodative paresis, blurred vision at distance from tonic accommodation, and light sensitivity from mydriasis.[15] Most symptoms will improve with time.

Patients with Adie's tonic pupil will typically present with a dilated pupil and anisocoria that is most apparent in bright illumination. The light response is sluggish or absent. The near response is better, although also sluggish with a slow redilation on return to distance fixation. On slit lamp examination, the pupil has an irregular shape with flattened areas of the pupil margin reflecting sectorial paralysis of the iris sphincter (Color Plate 2). The normal areas of the pupillary margin can be seen to contract on light stimulation, drawing nonreactive segments toward responsive segments. Although this finding is characteristic of Adie's syndrome, it is not pathognomonic, as similar observations are seen with other types of pupil abnormalities, including all of the tonic pupils.[16]

Accommodative Changes Accommodative paresis results from involvement of the ciliary body, and although initially most apparent, tends to improve with time. Tonic accommodation results in complaints of blurred distance vision and tends to be a later finding. Sectorial involvement of the ciliary body often results in an induced astigmatism at near.

Denervation Supersensitivity (Cholinergic Supersensitivity)
Postganglionic denervation typically results in supersensitivity of the iris sphincter to cholinergic drugs. The drug of choice to test for such supersensitivity is pilocarpine. Solutions of 0.125% and 0.1% are both appropriate. Neither concentration is available commercially and must be diluted in the office from commercial solutions. Therefore, although either concentration is appropriate, the 0.1% solution is easier to derive from a 1% pilocarpine solution.

Cholinergic sensitivity can be assessed using the following procedure:

1. Eliminate any residual miosis from a previous tonic near reaction by fogging the patient with plus lenses for 5 minutes.

2. Measure both pupils with a pupil gauge.
3. Instill two drops of 0.1% pilocarpine to each eye, separated by 30 seconds. The normal eye is used as a control.
4. Remeasure both pupils under the same lighting conditions after 30 minutes.

Do not allow the patient to sleep, read, or perform any task that might stimulate accommodation and falsify the results. The test for cholinergic supersensitivity as originally described[17] calls for photographing the pupils in different levels of room lighting before and after testing. Although this would more accurately document test results and is certainly more precise, measurements with a pupil gauge are more practical for the primary care clinician, who has an infrequent need to perform the test.

Diminished Corneal Sensation Because the sensory supply from the cornea travels through the ciliary ganglion via the short ciliary nerves, a lesion in either of these two places is likely to impair corneal sensation. Because the loss of corneal sensation is patchy,[18] a cotton wisp stroked across the eye will likely miss a focal area of sensation loss. Instead, corneal sensation should be tested with a focal stimulus such as a Cochet-Bonnet esthesiometer, which consists of a nylon filament that can be lengthened or shortened to provide a light or heavy touch (Figure 2.12). By varying the sensitivity, the corneal sensation can be mea-

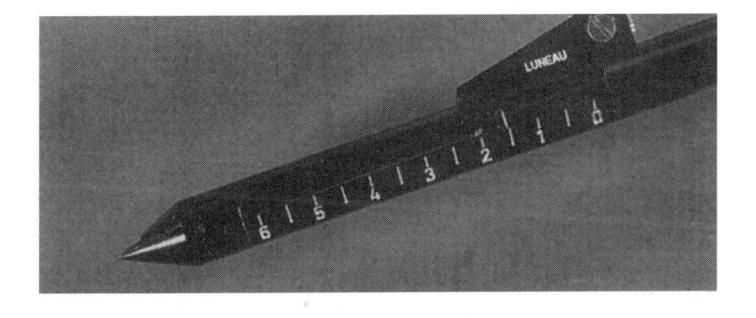

Figure 2.12 Cochet-Bonnet esthesiometer. (Reprinted with permission from CJ Cakanac, PC Ajamian. Cornea and Conjunctiva: Clinical Procedures. Boston: Butterworth–Heinemann, 1996;104.)

sured and recorded in areas of the cornea that correspond to clock hours. The corneal sensitivity is compared between the two eyes. If an esthesiometer is unavailable, focal stimulation is best accomplished with a tissue twisted to a point.

Diminished Tendon Reflexes Approximately 90% of the patients with Adie's tonic pupil have a benign hyporeflexia or areflexia of the tendon reflexes.[19] It should be emphasized that these patients are otherwise healthy and without any other evidence of autonomic or peripheral nervous system disease, distinguishing them from the neuropathic tonic pupil group. Testing the tendon reflexes is discussed in Chapter 4.

■ The Pupil in Midbrain Disease

Bilateral, mid-dilated, light-near dissociated pupils can be observed in patients with lesions in the dorsal midbrain in the region of the posterior commissure. The pupils are round and sluggish or unresponsive to light with an intact near response. The pupil abnormality is often the presenting sign of compressive disease in this area. Other signs may include supranuclear vertical gaze palsy, papilledema, convergence retraction nystagmus, fourth nerve palsy, and bilateral eyelid retraction (Collier's sign). Tumors of the pineal gland that expand to compress the dorsal midbrain are important causes of the dorsal midbrain syndrome (also known as *Parinaud's syndrome* or *sylvian aqueduct syndrome*). Other causes include hydrocephalus, infarction, hemorrhage, trauma, or infection in this area. The pupils can be distinguished from tonic pupils by their regular shape, brisk near response, and other associated features already mentioned.

Miotic, irregular pupils exhibiting light-near dissociation secondary to tertiary syphilis are to be distinguished from neuropathic tonic pupils secondary to syphilis. The former, Argyll-Robertson pupil, has irregular margins and no light response. Unlike the neuropathic tonic pupil, this is an extremely miotic pupil with a brisk near response. It is also bilateral and the lesion is thought to be in the rostral mesencephalon in the region of the sylvian aqueduct.[20] The miosis is presumed to be the result of interference of supranuclear inhibitory fibers as they approach the oculomotor nuclei.[20]

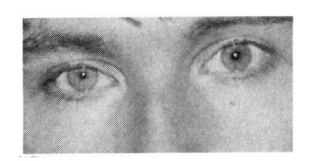

Figure 2.13
A patient with a right Horner's syndrome in bright illumination (A) and dim illumination (B). Note that the anisocoria is more readily observed in dim illumination.

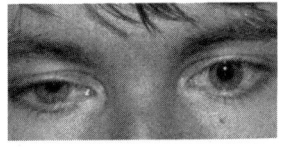

■ Horner's Syndrome

The oculosympathetic pathway can be interrupted at any location from its origin in the hypothalamus to its culmination in the orbit. The result is a Horner's syndrome characterized by ptosis, miosis, and facial anhydrosis. The ptosis of Horner's syndrome (Color Plate 3) is typically mild and results from paresis of Müller's muscle. The miosis occurs from paresis of the iris dilator and the resulting anisocoria is therefore more apparent in dim illumination (Figure 2.13). Despite the pupillary miosis, responses to light and near are intact. Reduced or absent facial sweating is characteristic of preganglionic Horner's syndrome—that is, interruption of sympathetics prior to the superior cervical ganglion. Recall that sympathetics controlling facial sweating reach the face via the external carotid artery. Fibers also travel with the internal carotid artery that control sweating to a small area of the face above the eyebrow. Therefore, a postganglionic Horner's syndrome may be characterized by loss of sweating above the brow.

Diagnosis of Horner's Syndrome

Although clinical diagnosis of Horner's syndrome is based on the clinical triad of ptosis, miosis, and anhydrosis, findings of inverse ptosis and dilation lag are useful diagnostic signs.

Inverse Ptosis Because sympathetics also control inferior eyelid musculature involved in retraction of the lower eyelid, when the

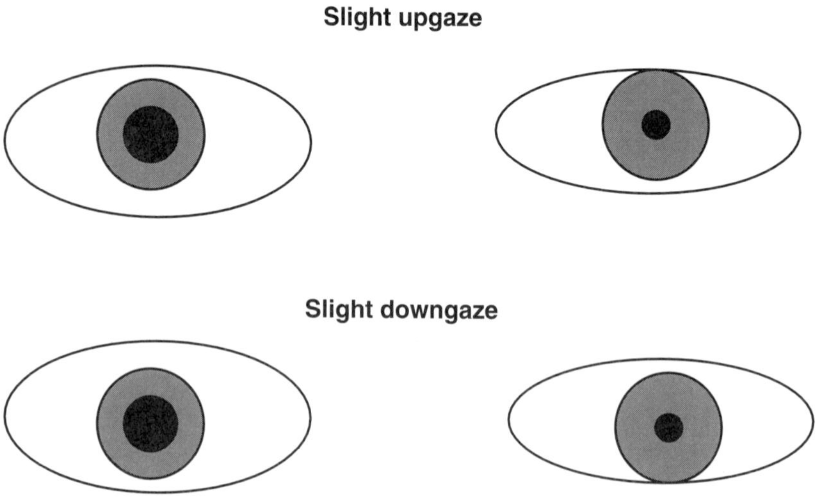

Slight upgaze

Slight downgaze

Figure 2.14 Schematic diagram depicting inverse ptosis of the left eye. In slight upgaze, there is sclera visible between the lower eyelids and limbus in both eyes. The patient slowly shifts gaze downward until the Horner's eye just touches the lower limbus. If sclera remains visible in the fellow eye, inverse ptosis is confirmed.

sympathetic supply is interrupted, the lower lid may become slightly elevated, and combined with the upper lid ptosis, gives the eye an enophthalmic appearance. Inverse ptosis is very subtle and is best seen by observing the inferior limbus as the patient follows a test object from slight upgaze toward downgaze. When the lower lid of the Horner's eye just touches the limbus, observation of the fellow eye will show sclera visible between the lower lid and limbus[21] (Figure 2.14).

Dilation Lag The anisocoria in Horner's syndrome is greatest in dim illumination when the loss of function of the dilator becomes more apparent. Anisocoria is also more readily observed immediately after room lights are dimmed, with the anisocoria becoming less apparent after 10–15 seconds.[22] Documenting this dilation lag can be done by photographing the pupils 4–5 seconds after the lights are turned off and then repeating the procedure 10–15 seconds after the lights are turned off (Figure 2.15).[23]

5 Seconds

15 Seconds

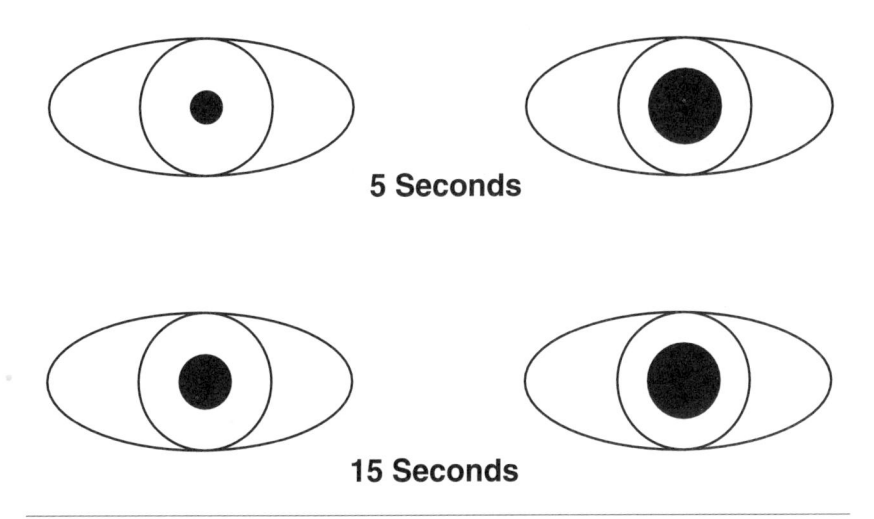

Figure 2.15 Schematic of dilation lag in Horner's syndrome. Note that the anisocoria is more apparent 5 seconds into darkness than it is after 15 seconds.

Pharmacologic Diagnosis Although strong clinical suspicion can be established using the above signs, confirmation is done with topical cocaine solution. Cocaine dilates normal pupils by blocking the reuptake of norepinephrine, the sympathetic neurotransmitter. Norepinephrine then accumulates at the receptor site, resulting in mydriasis. When the sympathetic pathway is interrupted, there is little or no physiologic release of norepinephrine; therefore, little or no accumulation occurs and little or no pupillary dilation results. A solution ranging from 4% to 10% of cocaine is adequate for pharmacologic diagnosis; the higher concentrations work faster.

Horner's syndrome can be confirmed pharmacologically using the following procedure:

1. Measure the pupils with a pupil gauge.
2. Instill two drops of solution of 4–10% cocaine into each eye separated by 5 minutes. The normal eye is used as a control.
3. Repeat pupillary measurements in 45 minutes. Horner's syndrome is confirmed if the normal eye dilates more than the suspect eye. The test is also considered positive if the anisocoria increases by more than 0.8 mm after the instillation of cocaine.[24]

The use of cocaine has drawbacks:

1. Cocaine is a poor mydriatic agent in patients with darkly pigmented irides and therefore has limited testing use for black patients.[25]
2. Because cocaine is a controlled substance, it is often not available to optometrists.
3. Patients who undergo cocaine testing will show traces in their urine for at least 36 hours after testing,[26] an important occupational consideration for those persons required to undergo drug screenings.

When cocaine testing is not applicable, the dilation lag becomes the most important diagnostic tool.

Localizing the Lesion in Horner's Syndrome

Pharmacologic testing with 1% hydroxyamphetamine solution localizes the lesion in Horner's syndrome to the preganglionic or postganglionic portion of the three-neuron pathway (Table 2.2). Hydroxyamphetamine is an indirect-acting sympathomimetic that works by releasing norepinephrine from postganglionic, sympathetic nerve terminals. When the central or preganglionic neurons are interrupted, hydroxyamphetamine will dilate the pupil because the postganglionic neuron is intact. In postganglionic Horner's syndrome, however, there is little or no norepinephrine in the nerve terminal, and the pupil fails to dilate.

Table 2.2 Summary of Localizing Features of Horner's Syndrome

	Cocaine	Hydroxyamphetamine	1% Phenylephrine	Sweat Pattern
First-order ("central")	No dilation	Dilation	No dilation	Entire half of body
Second-order ("intermediate," "preganglionic")	No dilation	Dilation	No dilation	Whole face and neck
Third-order ("postganglionic")	No dilation	No dilation	Dilation	Possible brow only

The procedure for hydroxyamphetamine localization is as follows:

1. Measure both pupils with a pupil gauge.
2. Instill 1 drop of 1% hydroxyamphetamine solution into each eye. After 5 minutes, instill a second drop.
3. Measure pupil sizes under the same lighting conditions in 45 minutes.[27]

Dilation of the Horner's pupil localizes the lesion to the central or preganglionic portion of the sympathetic pathway. Failure to dilate localizes the lesion to the postganglionic or third-order neuron.

Denervation supersensitivity in Horner's syndrome is typically seen in postganglionic lesions. The best way to demonstrate denervation supersensitivity is with 1% phenylephrine solution, a direct-acting sympathomimetic. Instillation of one drop into each eye will show greater dilation in the Horner's eye if the lesion is postganglionic.[28]

Localizing lesions in Horner's syndrome is not limited to pharmacologic testing. Careful evaluation of clinical signs often provides useful localizing clues. For example, although it is not possible to distinguish a central from a preganglionic Horner's with hydroxyamphetamine, central lesions will rarely present without clinically apparent brainstem signs. Patients with preganglionic Horner's may have arm pain or a history of cardiothoracic surgery or neck surgery. Clinical localizing features of postganglionic Horner's include facial pain and evidence of cavernous sinus syndrome.

Sweating patterns may also provide valuable localizing clues. Patients with central Horner's may have ipsilateral loss of sweating on the entire half of the body. Patients with intermediate or preganglionic Horner's may have reduced or absent sweating of the ipsilateral face and neck. Patients with postganglionic Horner's often experience normal sweating, but there may be a disturbance in the ipsilateral brow area. Traditionally, confirmation of anhydrosis was done with quinizarin powder, a color indicator, but it is difficult to obtain,[29] and the frequency of its use limits its practicality. The simplest way to assess relative sweating on either side of the face or body is to compare the skin resistance with a smooth object rubbed against the skin, preferably after the patient becomes exerted. The author recommends the smooth side of a prism bar, which is lightly dragged across the skin (Figure 2.16). If sweating is reduced or absent, the prism bar will move across the skin with little resistance. If sweating is intact, the plastic will stick as it is dragged across the skin.

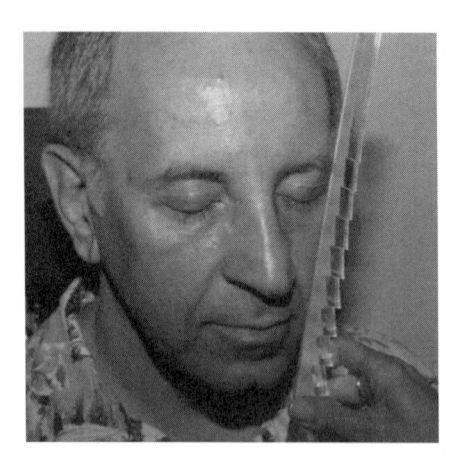

Figure 2.16
A clean, smooth object such as a prism bar can be dragged across the skin to assess sweating patterns in Horner's syndrome.

■ The Pupil in Third Nerve Palsy

Pupil involvement in third nerve palsy is characterized by pupillary dilation with a poor response to light and near. Pupil involvement is an important observation because pupillary involvement in the setting of acute third nerve palsy is presumed to be due to an aneurysm,[30] whereas pupil sparing in acute third nerve palsy is most likely due to infarction of the nerve fascicle.[31] The examiner must be aware, however, that aneurysmal third nerve palsies may present initially with pupil sparing, with the pupil becoming involved within 3–5 days.[32] In such cases, the palsy is typically incomplete, with pupillary involvement becoming apparent as the palsy evolves.

Unusual pupil behavior is also seen in aberrant third nerve regeneration after an acute third nerve palsy. After trauma to the nerve, anomalous reinnervation occurs with misdirection of axons supplying the various extraocular muscles and the pupil. The pupil findings in aberrant regeneration include a fixed (miotic or dilated) pupil with a sectorial response seen on slit lamp biomicroscopy. When eye movement occurs in a direction requiring third nerve input, the pupil constricts. This is especially true on attempted adduction. Pupil findings in aberrant regeneration are similar to those seen in tonic pupils and are differentiated by history, as well as by associated findings of limited motility. Eyelid retraction on downgaze and adduction are also commonly seen in aberrant third nerve regeneration. Although aberrant regeneration typically follows acute third nerve palsy, it is also seen in patients with slowly compressive lesions of the third nerve where there is no history of acute third nerve palsy.[33,34]

■ The Pupil in Pharmacologic Blockade

It is not unusual for a fixed, dilated pupil to occur from the accidental instillation of a mydriatic/cycloplegic agent without any recollection from the patient. Such pupils are fixed to light and near and are accompanied by accommodative paralysis. In most instances, careful history will reveal the source of the offending agent. The greatest fear among medical practitioners of all types is that the fixed pupil represents the initial presentation of an aneurysmal third nerve palsy. A fixed, dilated pupil in an otherwise healthy, ambulatory patient is rarely due to an intracranial aneurysm.[35] Furthermore, the possibility that a fixed pupil is due to a third nerve palsy in the absence of ptosis or any motility disturbance is extremely remote. Despite the improbability, the potential morbidity and mortality associated with intracranial aneurysm requires that such a condition be definitively ruled out. Unfortunately, the diagnostic tests that are necessary to rule out intracranial disease are not only expensive and time-consuming, but can also be harmful or even fatal to the patient. There is, however, a very simple test that can distinguish a pharmacologic pupil from other causes, namely, from mydriasis secondary to aneurysmal third nerve palsy. Instillation of one drop of 1% pilocarpine solution will constrict a normal pupil as well as a fixed, dilated pupil from a third nerve palsy or postganglionic denervation. It will not, however, budge a pupil that has been dilated with atropine or other anticholinergic drug.[36]

Billing and Reimbursement

Tests of pupil testing are included as part of a comprehensive eye examination, and there are no applicable separate Current Procedural Terminology codes. Performing pupil testing, however, may justify increasing the office visit code to a higher level.

■ Related International Classification of Diseases-9 (ICD-9) Terminology

Abnormal pupillary function	379.40
Anisocoria	379.41
Miosis (persistent)	379.42

Mydriasis (persistent)   379.43
Argyll-Robertson pupil   379.45
Tonic pupil   379.46
Horner's syndrome   337.9

■ References

1. Levatin P. Pupillary escape in disease of the retina or optic nerve. Arch Ophthalmol 1959;62:768–779.
2. Thompson HS. Light-near dissociation of the pupil. Ophthalmologica 1984;189:21–23.
3. Thompson HS. Afferent pupillary defects. Pupillary findings associated with defects of the afferent arm of the pupillary light reflex. Am J Ophthalmol 1966;62:860–873.
4. Browning DJ, Tiedemen JS. The test light affects quantitation of the afferent pupillary defect. Ophthalmology 1987;94:53–55.
5. Johnson LN. The effect of light intensity on measurement of the relative afferent pupillary defect. Am J Ophthalmol 1990;109:481–482.
6. Thompson HS. Pupillary signs in the diagnosis of optic nerve disease. Trans Ophthalmol Soc UK 1976;96:377–381.
7. Burde RM, Savino PJ, Trobe JD. Clinical Decisions in Neuro-Ophthalmology (2nd ed). St. Louis: Mosby, 1992.
8. Borchert M, Sadun AA. Bright light stimuli as a mask of relative afferent pupillary defects. Am J Ophthalmol 1988;106:98–99.
9. Thompson HS, Corbett JJ, Cox TA. How to measure the relative afferent pupillary defect. Surv Ophthalmol 1981;26:39–42.
10. Cox TA. Pupillary escape. Neurology 1992;42:1271–1276.
11. Bell RA, Waggoner PM, Boyd WM, et al. Clinical grading of relative afferent pupillary defects. Arch Ophthalmol 1993;111:938–942.
12. Johnson LN, Hill RA, Bartholomew MJ. Correlation of afferent pupillary defect with visual field loss on automated perimetry. Ophthalmology 1988;96:1649–1655.
13. Thompson HS, Montague P, Cox TA, Corbett JJ. The relationship between visual acuity, pupillary defect, and visual field loss. Am J Ophthalmol 1982;93:681–688.
14. Thompson HS. A Classification of "Tonic Pupils." In HS Thompson, R Dariff, L Frisen, et al. (eds), Topics in Neuro-Ophthalmology. Baltimore: Williams & Wilkins, 1979;94–95.
15. Bell RA, Thompson HS. The Symptoms of Adie's Syndrome. In HS Thompson, R Dariff, L Frisen, et al. (eds), Topics in Neuro-Ophthalmology. Baltimore: Williams & Wilkins, 1979;9–104.
16. Thompson HS. Segmental palsy of the iris sphincter. Arch Ophthalmol 1978;96:1615–1620.

17. Bourgon P, Pilley SFJ, Thompson HS. Cholinergic supersensitivity of the iris sphincter in Adie's tonic pupil. Am J Ophthalmol 1978;85:373–377.
18. Purcell JJ, Krachmer JH, Thompson HS. Corneal sensation in Adie's syndrome. Am J Ophthalmol 1977;84:496–500.
19. Thompson HS, Bourgon P, Van Allen MW. The Tendon Reflexes in Adie's Tonic Pupil. In HS Thompson, R Dariff, L Frisen, et al. (eds), Topics in Neuro-Ophthalmology. Baltimore: Williams & Wilkins, 1979;104–112.
20. Miller NR. Walsh and Hoyt's Clinical Neuro-Ophthalmology (4th ed). Baltimore: Williams & Wilkins, 1985;483–487.
21. Grimson BS, Thompson HS. Horner's Syndrome: Overall View of 120 Cases. In HS Thompson, R Dariff, L Frisen, et al. (eds), Topics in Neuro-Ophthalmology. Baltimore: Williams & Wilkins, 1979;151–156.
22. Pilley SFJ, Thompson HS. The pupillary dilation lag in Horner's syndrome. Br J Ophthalmol 1975;59:731–735.
23. van der Wiel HL, van Gijn J. Horner's syndrome: criteria for oculosympathetic denervation. J Neurol Sci 1982;56:293–298.
24. Kardon RH, Denison CG, Brown CK, et al. Critical evaluation of the cocaine test in the diagnosis of Horner's syndrome. Arch Ophthalmol 1990;108:384–387.
25. Friedman JR, Whiting DW, Kosmorsky GS, et al. The cocaine test in normal patients. Am J Ophthalmol 1984;98:808–810.
26. Bralliar BB, Skarf B, Owens JB. Ophthalmic use of cocaine and the urine test for benzoylergonine. N Engl J Med 1989;320:1757–1758.
27. Thompson HS, Mensher JH. Adrenergic mydriasis in Horner's syndrome. Hydroxyamphetamine for diagnosis of postganglionic dfects. Am J Ophthalmol 1971;72:472–480.
28. Grimson BS,Thompson HS. The Post-Ganglionic Horner's Syndrome. In JS Glaser (ed), Neuro-Ophthalmology, St. Louis: Mosby, 1975;Vol. 9, 190–198; Vol. 8, 265–270.
29. Myles WM. Oh, let's just do this simple test! Can J Ophthalmol 1994;Feb 29: 43–44.
30. Rucker CW. The causes of paralysis of the third, fourth and sixth cranial nerves. Am J Ophthalmol 1958;46:787–794.
31. Goldstein JE, Cogan DG. Diabetic ophthalmoplegia with special reference to the pupil. Arch Ophthalmol 1960;64:592–600.
32. Kissel JT, Burde RM, Klingele TG, et al. Pupil-sparing oculomotor palsies with internal carotid-posterior communicating artery aneurysms. Ann Neurol 1983;13:149–154.
33. Johnson LN, Kamper CA, Hepler RS, et al. Primary aberrant regeneration of the oculomotor nerve from presumed extracavernous neurilemmoma, meningioma, and asymmetric mammillary body. Neuro-Ophthalmology 1989;9:227–232.
34. Cox TA, Wurster JB, Godfrey WA. Primary aberrant oculomotor regeneration due to intracranial aneurysm. Arch Neurol 1979;36:570–571.
35. Payne JW, Adamkiewicz J Jr. Unilateral internal ophthalmoplegia with intracranial aneurysm: report of a case. Am J Ophthalmol 1969;68:349–352.
36. Thompson HS, Newsome DA, Loewenfeld IE. The fixed dilated pupil: sudden iridoplegia or mydriatic drugs? A simple diagnostic test. Arch Ophthal 1971;86:21–27.

Color Plate 1
Hyperemic extraocular muscle insertion and conjunctival hyperemia in a patient with Graves' orbitopathy. (Reprinted with permission from JJ Kanski. The Eye in Systemic Disease [2nd ed]. Oxford: Butterworth–Heinemann, 1990;13.)

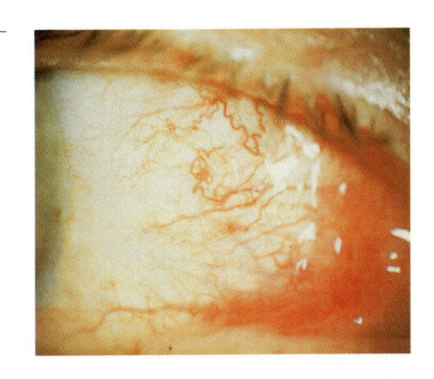

Color Plate 2
Irregular pupil margins with flattened areas reflect sector paralysis in this patient with tonic pupil.

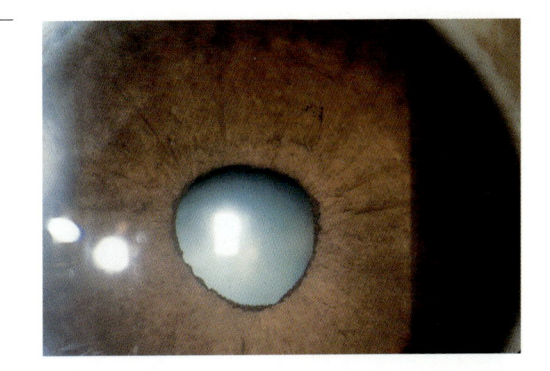

Color Plate 3
Iris heterochromia in a patient with congenital Horner's syndrome.

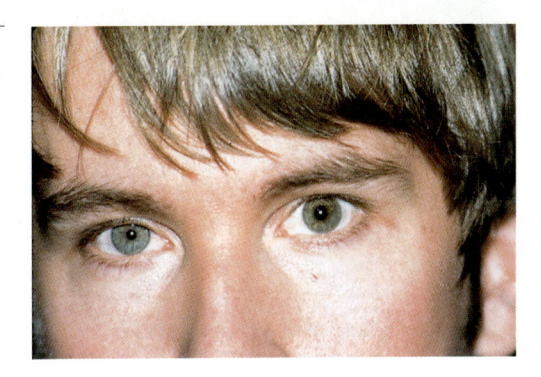

Color Plate 4
Test stimuli for tangent screen visual field testing are available in different sizes and colors.

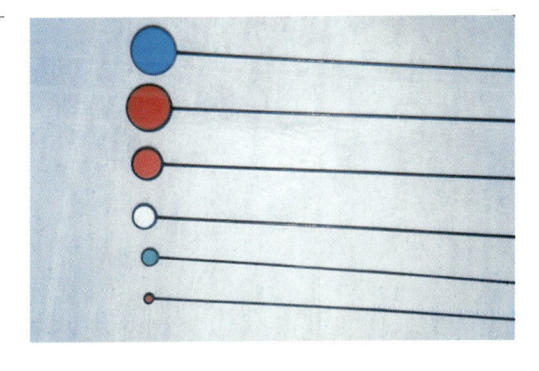

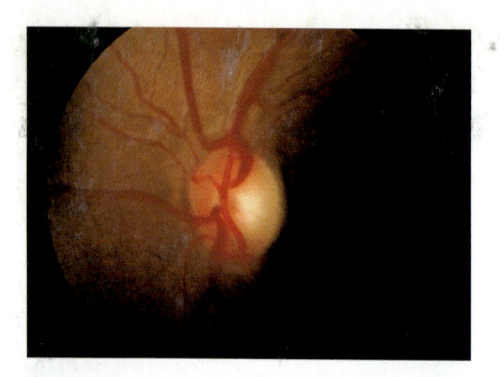

Color Plate 5
Temporal pallor of the optic nerve in alcohol-related nutritional optic neuropathy.

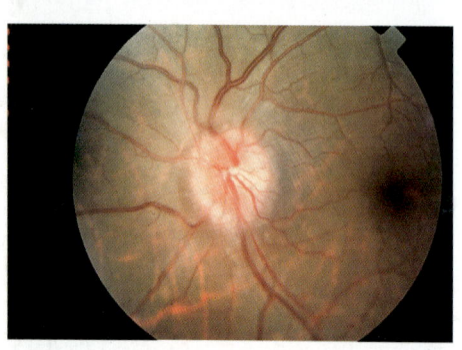

Color Plate 6
Disc edema in a patient with optic neuritis.

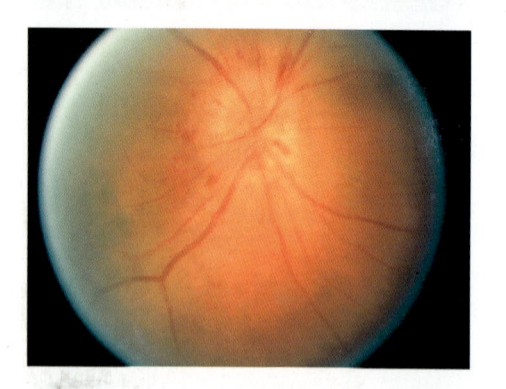

Color Plate 7
Disc edema and flame hemorrhages in a patient with anterior ischemic optic neuropathy.

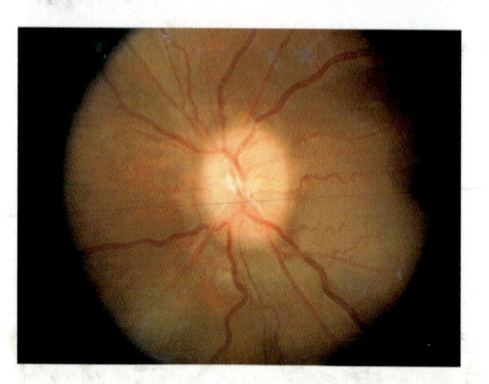

Color Plate 8
Papilledema in a patient with pseudotumor cerebri.

Color Plate 9
Drusen of the optic nerve.

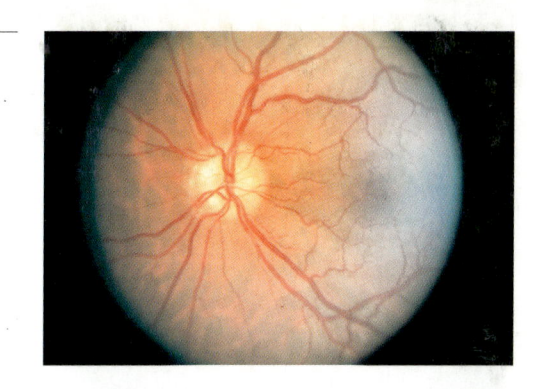

Color Plate 10
Optic nerve hypoplasia with a peripapillary halo, or "double ring sign."

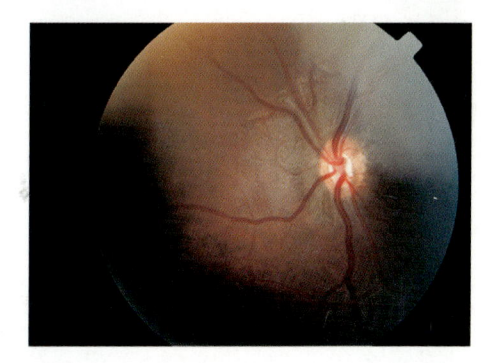

Color Plate 11
Optic nerve coloboma.

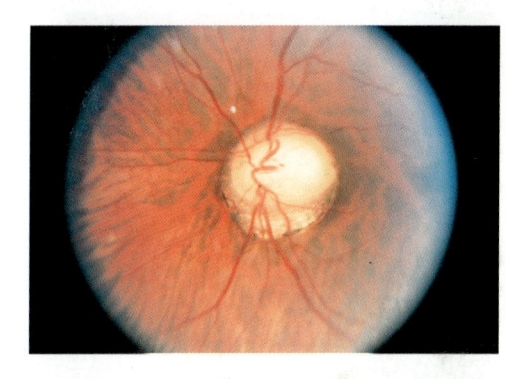

Color Plate 12
Optic pit.

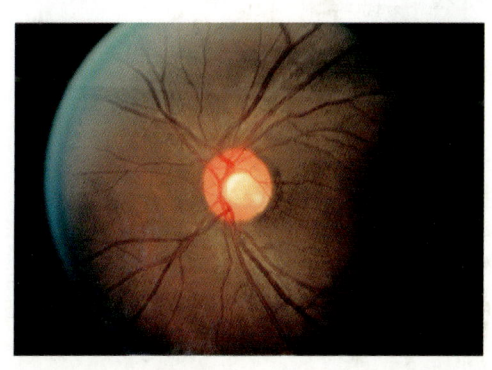

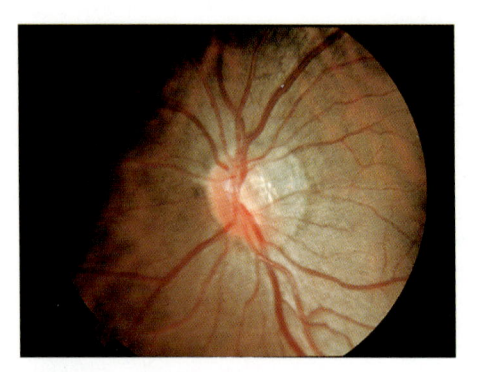

Color Plate 13
Tilted disc.

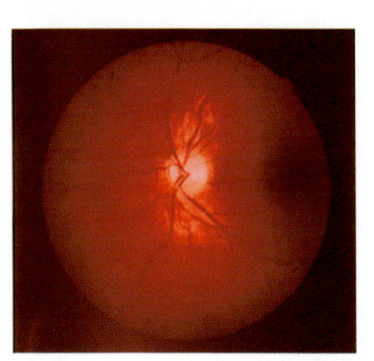

Color Plate 14
Left optic nerve in a patient with a right optic tract lesion. Note that the disc pallor is most apparent nasally and temporally, forming a band pattern.

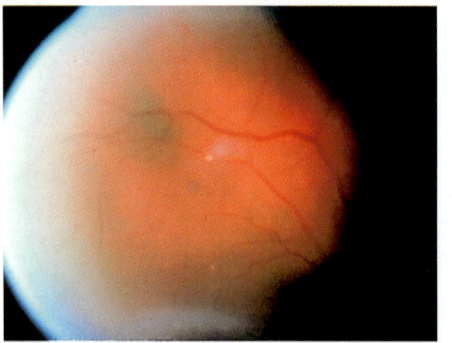

Color Plate 15
Retinal embolus in a patient with carotid occlusive disease.

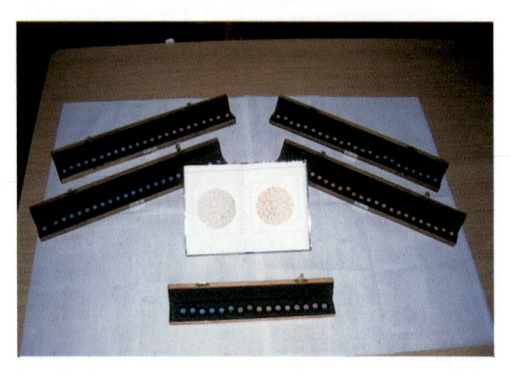

Color Plate 16
Tests of color vision. Pseudo-isochromatic plates (center), Farnsworth-Munsell 100-Hue (back) and Panel D-15 (front).

3

Visual Field Evaluation in Neuro-Ophthalmic Disease

The visual field is a topographic representation of the visual pathway from its origin at the retinal photoreceptors to its culmination in the visual cortex of the occipital lobe. Visual stimuli travel through the ocular media to the retina. After being processed by retinal photoreceptors, retinal ganglion cells transport information to the optic nerves, whose axons are a continuation of the retinal ganglion cells. In the optic chiasm, nasal fibers representing the temporal visual field cross, and the temporal fibers representing nasal visual field do not cross. Therefore, once fibers reach the optic tract, the fibers representing the right half of the visual field are located in the left visual pathway, and those representing the left half of the visual field are located in the right visual pathway. After crossing in the chiasm, fibers travel in the optic tract to the lateral geniculate bodies. From there, the optic radiations (geniculocalcarine radiations) loop forward and inferiorly in the temporal lobe before traveling posteriorly through the temporal and parietal lobes, ultimately reaching area 17 of the occipital cortex.

Visual field testing is a vital aspect of neuro-ophthalmic system evaluation. The purpose of visual field analysis in neuro-ophthalmic disease is threefold. The first purpose is to detect any abnormality, whether focal or general, in the hill of vision; the second is to localize the pathology in the visual pathway; and the third is to quantitatively document the defect so that progression or improvement in response to treatment can be monitored.

With the growing sophistication of perimetric equipment, visual field assessment has become rather complex and expensive. For this reason, it is not prudent to do formal visual field testing on each patient. Rather, a strategy to identify those patients who are more likely to have visual field defects should be used. Such an approach begins with the case history that often reveals clues to whether a visual field defect exists. It is not unusual for patients with visual field defects to report reduced vision in one or both eyes. This is true of disease of the optic nerves, chiasm, or occipital lobe tip. Patients with complete bitemporal hemianopia may report difficulty with peripheral or central vision and, rarely, diplopia due to an unstable overlap of defective visual fields.[1] Patients with right homonymous hemianopia will report difficulty reading despite normal visual acuity, whereas those with left homonymous hemianopia will report frequent loss of place when reading from one line to the next. Patients with bitemporal and right or left homonymous hemianopia may report mobility problems, clumsiness, or frequent falls or perhaps some accidents or close calls when engaged in such tasks as operating a motor vehicle or crossing the street. If patients deny visual field–related difficulty, questioning close friends or family members may reveal signs of mobility disturbance or behavior suggestive of neurologic disease. In visual field defects that are the result of disease in the brain or its associations, neurologic deficits or related symptomatology may be apparent. Finally, patients with known head injury or other neurologic disease are more likely to exhibit visual field defects.

In addition to clues in the history, a number of other important examination features may alert clinicians to the possibility that a visual field defect exists. Simply observing how a patient reads the acuity chart (subjective Snellen acuity) is often very helpful. Patients with hemianopic visual field defects often have difficulty reading the side of the chart that corresponds to the visual field defect. Patients with altitudinal defects or central scotomas will often report that they can see more clearly when they look eccentrically. This behavior may also be observed by the examiner as the patient struggles to find the eye position that facilitates vision. Other important examination findings that may be apparent include color vision abnormalities, reduced visual acuity, and the presence of an afferent pupillary defect.

The visual field is defined as "that portion in space that is visible to the steadily fixating eye."[2] The extent of the visual field in normals is determined by eyelid position and facial contours. In normal individuals, it extends 60 degrees nasally, 90 degrees temporally, 50 degrees superiorly, and 70 degrees inferiorly.[3] The visual field has its greatest sensitivity at the point corresponding to the fovea. From there, it drops off quickly within 10 degrees of fixation and then tapers steadily before losing sensitivity dramatically in the periphery. The overall sensitivity of the visual field can be depicted as a three-dimensional structure with the highest point corresponding to the fovea.[4] Defects in the visual field consist of depressions, both diffuse or focal, in any part of the hill of vision, and perimetry is a means by which clinicians detect these changes.

The prerequisite to the undertaking of any formal visual field study is the confrontation visual field. Confrontation visual fields are useful in the identification of visual field defects before formal testing and in introducing the patient to visual field skills. As a screening examination, confrontation visual fields are limited in their ability to detect small defects seen in early disease processes, but central scotomas, altitudinal defects, and hemianopic defects, all common in neurologic disease, are readily detected. When performed carefully and correctly, confrontation testing can be extremely sensitive while remaining rapid, making it an ideal screening tool. It is also a valuable tool for patients who are unable to perform or respond to formal perimetric techniques because of age or physical or cognitive limitations.

The best approach to confrontation testing involves static presentation of targets in the central portion of the visual field. It is inappropriate to present a moving stimulus from the periphery because movement can easily be perceived in the far periphery and dense central defects without peripheral extension will likely be missed. The vast majority of visual field defects seen in neuro-ophthalmic disease involve the central 30 degrees of visual field, and this is the area that is closely investigated in confrontation visual field testing.

Method for Confrontation Visual Field Testing

The patient and examiner are seated facing each other approximately 50 cm apart. Testing is done monocularly, with the patient covering either eye with the palm of his or her hand (covering with fingers is unacceptable because it may be possible for the patient to see through the spaces). The patient fixates the examiner's nose for the duration of the test. The field is divided into four quadrants defined by the vertical and horizontal hemianopic lines. The horizontal hemianopic line divides the visual field into superior and inferior halves and is anatomically determined by the superior and inferior arcuate bundles. The vertical hemianopic line separates the right and left halves of the visual field and is determined anatomically by the separation of nasal and temporal pathway fibers at the optic chiasm. The nose provides a nice fixation point, which divides the face into right and left halves as well as upper and lower halves. Uniform room lighting is essential for accurate results. Basic confrontation visual field testing is divided into four parts: finger counting, simultaneous finger counting, simultaneous hand comparison, and comparison of colored targets.

■ Finger Counting

Fingers are presented vertically in one quadrant at a time at a distance midway between examiner and patient and approximately 3 inches from the midline. It is best to present one, two, or five fingers oriented vertically to minimize patient confusion. The patient is asked to report the number of fingers present. Very young children and nonverbal or demented adults can be asked to mimic the number of fingers presented, or the examiner can simply watch for eye movement elicited by the stimulus. If the examiner desires, gross testing of the peripheral field can be done by presenting fingers at shoulder width and beyond.

■ Simultaneous Finger Counting

Holding the hands 6 inches apart, the examiner simultaneously presents fingers in two opposite quadrants on either side of the vertical hemianopic line (Figure 3.1). Simultaneous comparison of nasal and temporal quadrants may demonstrate a subtler defect that could not be demonstrated by individual quadrant testing. Even more important, it is used to test for the extinction phenomenon, which is seen in parietal lobe disease and causes the patient to ignore one side of the visual field.[5]

■ Simultaneous Hand Comparison

The examiner places one hand in the nasal and one hand in the temporal half of the patient's field. The patient is asked if one hand is darker, blur-

Figure 3.1
Simultaneous finger counting in confrontation visual field testing. The examiner is seated approximately 50 cm away from the patient. Presentation of fingers is about shoulder width or 6 inches apart.

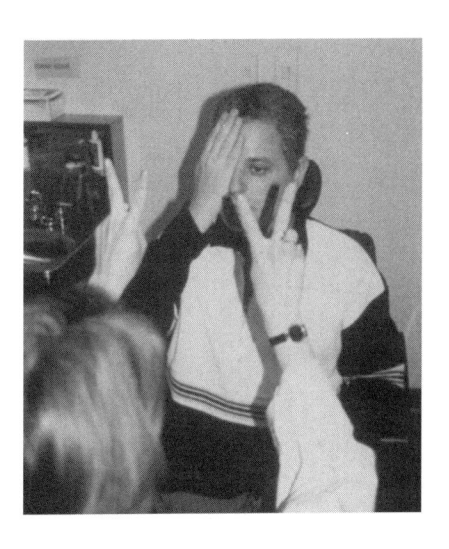

rier, or more difficult to see than the other while maintaining fixation on the nose. The same is done across the horizontal hemianopic line to compare the upper and lower halves of the visual field. Simultaneous comparison of targets helps to elicit relative defects in the visual field that are too subtle to be discovered by single quadrant stimulation.

■ Comparison of Colored Targets

Field defects that occur in the pregeniculate visual pathway are often more sensitive to red stimuli.[6] Using red targets can therefore enhance detection of lesions in the optic nerves, chiasm, and optic tracts. The examiner presents a red object in any two quadrants and asks the patient to report any difference in the color saturation in one quadrant relative to another (Figure 3.2). If a difference is noted, a relative defect exists, and the extent can be plotted by moving the stimulus into or out of the field defect and asking the patient to report when the color changes. Red targets can also be used to detect relative central or cecocentral scotomas by placing one test object centrally and one paracentrally and asking the patient to compare the two.

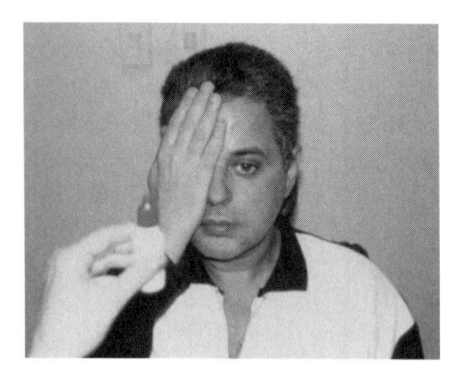

Figure 3.2
Comparison of colored targets using the red caps of mydriatic bottles.

Manual Perimetry

The mainstay of manual perimetry is the Goldmann perimeter. Generally speaking, the Goldmann perimeter is a bowl perimeter that uses a kinetic approach to visual field testing, that is, moving targets are presented from the periphery. There are six stimulus sizes indicated by Roman numerals. To control stimulus intensity, a coarse adjustment system in 0.5 log unit increments is indicated by Arabic numbers. A fine adjustment in 0.1 log unit increments is designated with Arabic letters.

Goldmann perimetry has fallen off in popularity because it cannot match the threshold capabilities of automated perimetry to evaluate and monitor glaucomatous visual field defects. Such defects make up the greatest percentage of visual fields done in the majority of eye care settings. Automated perimetry has also become the test of choice in the detection and monitoring of patients with neuro-ophthalmic visual field defects; however, manual perimetry remains useful in evaluating those patients who are physically or cognitively incapable of performing an automated test. Goldmann perimetry also has a distinct advantage over automated perimetry because it can quickly determine the extent of the peripheral visual field.

■ Performing the Test

At least two isopters are typically plotted in Goldmann perimetry. The size I stimulus is the smallest available, and this is generally an appropriate starting point for most individuals. Larger stimulus sizes are used only when vision is not adequate to see smaller stimuli. The test is performed as follows:

1. The instrument is calibrated. The perimeter is equipped with a calibrating device and instructions.
2. The paper is inserted into the designated compartment, and the notched markings are aligned with the designated notches on the instrument. Tightening the designated knobs will firmly lock the paper in place.
3. Testing is done monocularly. The patient is positioned in the instrument and the eye to be tested is aligned.
4. The examiner starts with the I2e isopter by choosing the corresponding numbers and letter on the control panel.
5. The stimulus is moved radially from nonseeing parts of the periphery toward fixation. A speed of 4 degrees per second has been determined to be optimal for testing the peripheral field.[7]
6. The patient is instructed to signal the examiner when the stimulus is seen, and the examiner marks the corresponding point on the recording sheet. This is repeated at regular intervals throughout the periphery, and the points are then connected to mark the corresponding isopter.
7. The I4e isopter is plotted next. Less intense isopters should also be plotted when clinical suspicion that a defect exists is strong. When testing the central 30 degrees of the visual field, an appropriate near correction should be placed in its designated holder.
8. Once the isopters are plotted, static spot-checking at several locations within each isopter is done to look for scotomas. If a scotoma is detected, threshold concepts can then be applied to measure the depth of the scotoma by gradually increasing the stimulus intensity until it is seen. The fine adjustment is useful here. The size of the scotoma is recorded by moving the stimulus from within the scotoma outward from nonseeing to seeing. Repeating this with different intensities will determine the slope of the defect (Figure 3.3).

■ Goldmann Approach to Neuro-Ophthalmic Visual Field Defects

Neuro-ophthalmologic visual field defects are frequently characterized by their respect for the vertical or horizontal hemianopic lines. Such

NEURO-OPHTHALMIC SYSTEM: CLINICAL PROCEDURES

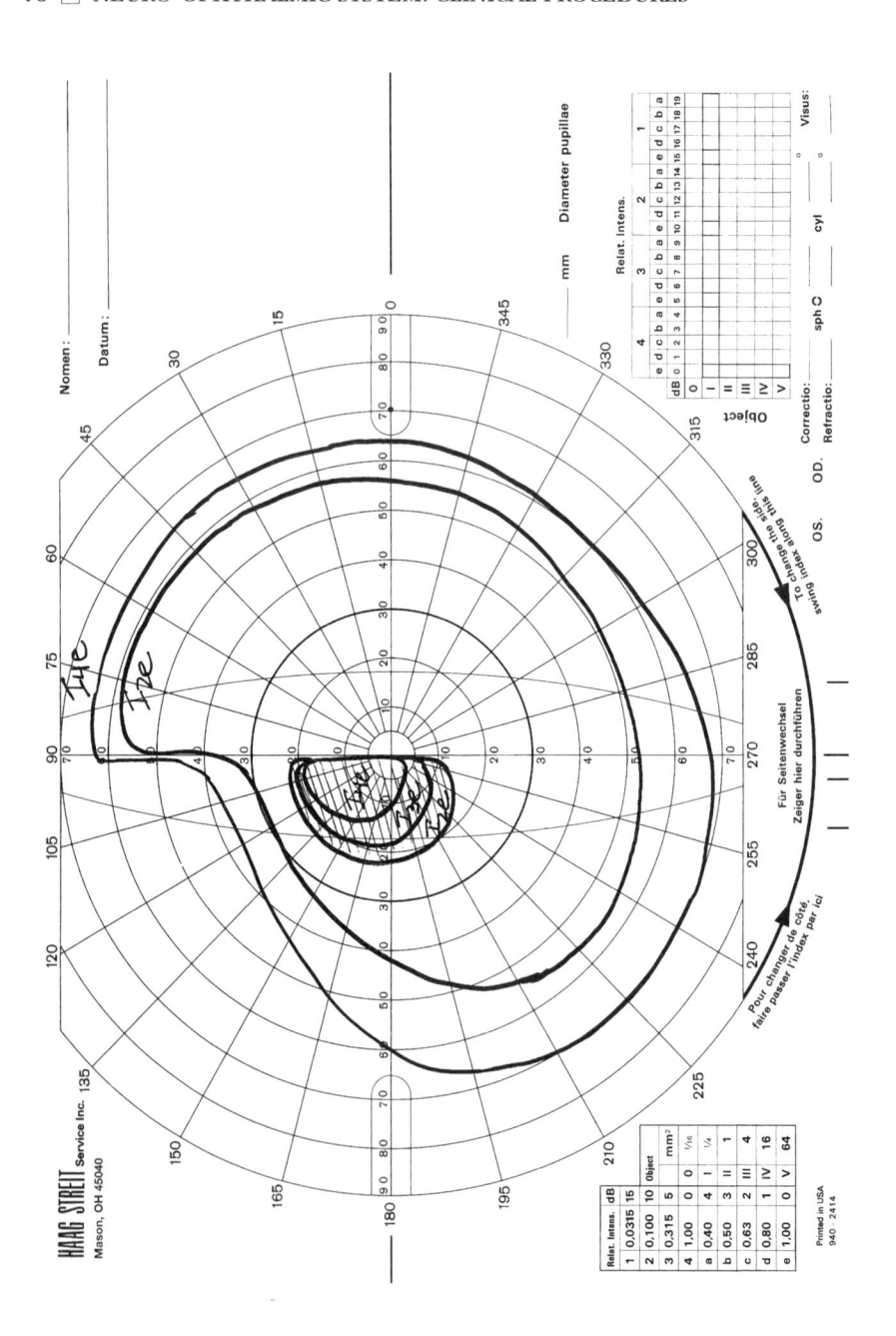

◀ **Figure 3.3** Superior temporal depression in the left eye with a central temporal dense scotoma. Note that the edge has a steep margin at the midline and a sloping margin at the remaining edges.

defects can be investigated selectively by paying close attention to the vertical hemianopic line or, put simply, that line that separates the right and left sides of the visual field. Such defects respect the vertical hemianopic line—that is, they lie on one side or the other without crossing over. The same is true of defects that respect the horizontal hemianopic line or horizontal raphe. The Goldmann approach is as follows:

1. To investigate hemianopic visual field defects, the examiner begins in the periphery 5–10 degrees from the vertical hemianopic line and moves the stimulus inward and parallel to the vertical hemianopic line (Figure 3.4A). The same is repeated on the other side of the vertical hemianopic line.
2. A vertical step occurs when there is a difference in where the patient sees the stimulus. When such a step occurs, the hemianopic line should then be approached perpendicularly to confirm respect for the vertical hemianopic line (Figure 3.4B).
3. Finally, static spot-checking not only checks for scotomas within the isopter but also further confirms the hemianopic defect.
4. Stronger stimuli can then be used in a selective fashion to quantify the defect.
5. The same principles can be applied when investigating defects that respect the horizontal raphe.

One drawback to the kinetic approach to neuro-ophthalmic visual field defects is the Riddoch phenomenon.[8,9] Such a phenomenon occurs within a hemianopic field defect when the stimulus is seen when moving but is not seen when presented statically. This makes it difficult to plot out isopters accurately, and the patient is often mislabeled as inconsistent. If there appears to be a marked difference in the visibility between moving and nonmoving stimuli, it is best to quantify the visual field defect using a static approach.

Figure 3.4 ▶ (A) To determine whether a vertical hemianopic defect exists, the stimulus is moved parallel to the vertical hemianopic line on either side. A vertical step exists when there is a difference in where the stimulus is seen on one side relative to the other. (B) Approaching the hemianopic line perpendicularly from nonseeing confirms the existence of the defect.

78 □ NEURO-OPHTHALMIC SYSTEM: CLINICAL PROCEDURES

A

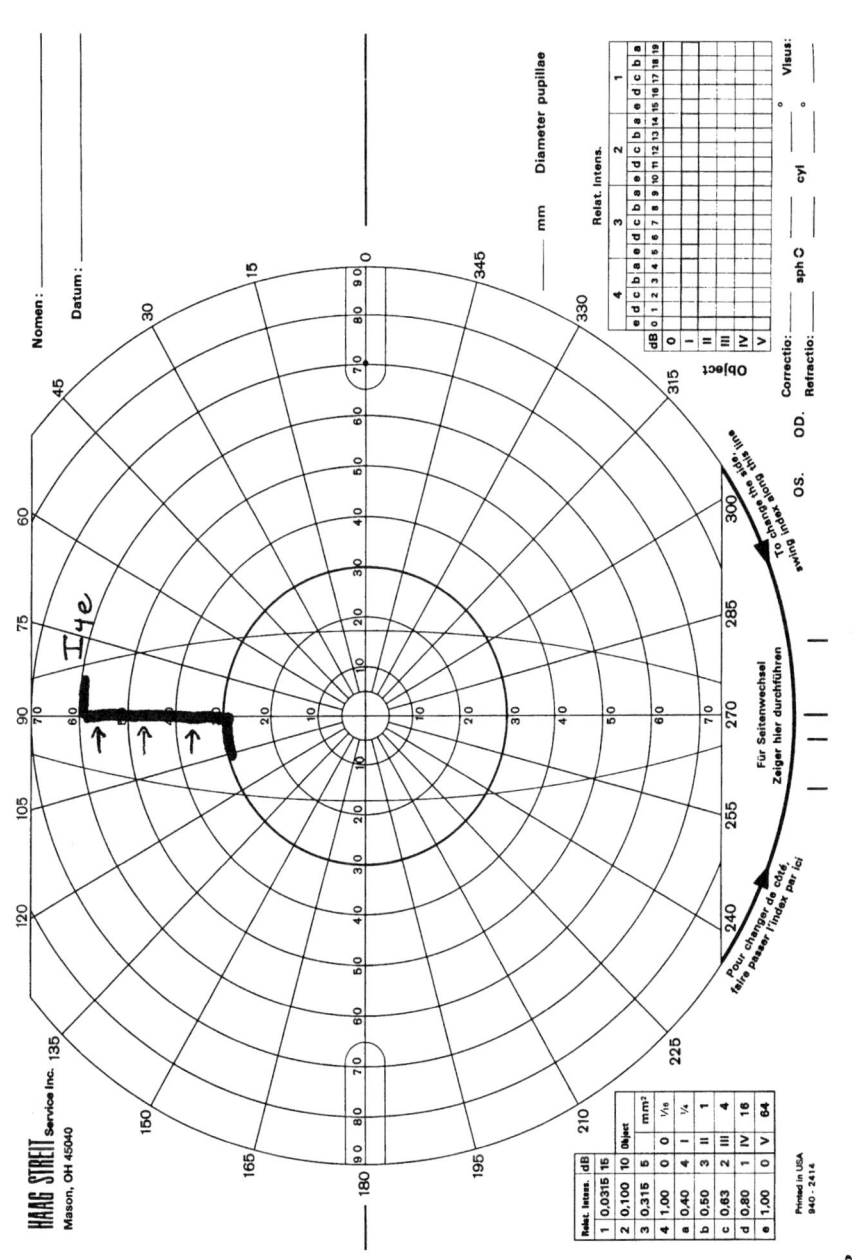

Visual Field Evaluation in Neuro-Ophthalmic Disease □ **79**

B

Tangent Screen

Although tangent screen visual field testing is considered by many to be obsolete, it has an important place in neuro-ophthalmic disease. It is a useful alternative to both Goldmann and automated perimetry, especially when a patient cannot access the perimeter bowl, as is frequently the case in patients with debilitating neurologic disease. Test distances can be varied, a useful option in patients with functional visual field defects (i.e., malingering and hysteria). At a test distance of 1 m, the tangent screen measures the central 30 degrees of the visual field, an area most often involved in neuro-ophthalmic disease.

The tangent screen consists of a square black cloth with stitching to show the position of the blind spot, delineate quadrants, and mark the distance from fixation at 5-degree increments. Test stimuli vary in size and are available in white, blue, red, and green colors (Color Plate 4). They can be interchanged on long, black wands that match the background of the screen. Visual field testing is done much the same way as in Goldmann except that only the stimulus size can be varied, not the intensity.

The method for tangent screen testing is as follows:

1. The patient is seated 1 m from the screen. The left eye is patched, and the patient is instructed to fixate on a centrally located fixation target.
2. The examiner should begin with the smallest stimulus the patient is able to see, reserving larger sizes for those patients who are unable to see the smaller sizes.
3. The stimulus is moved inward at a speed of approximately 5 degrees per second.
4. The patient is instructed to verbally signal the examiner when the stimulus is observed.
5. Response locations are marked on the screen with black-headed pins that blend into the background of the screen. When testing is completed, the pin locations are marked on the recording sheet, and the points are connected to form isopters. The color and size of the stimulus are also noted on the recording sheet.

As in confrontation visual field testing, the use of colored targets (particularly red) increases test sensitivity in neuro-ophthalmic disease. When using red targets, the patient is instructed to signal the examiner when the stimulus color is recognized. Likewise, when a defect is noted, its extent can be quantitated by moving the stimulus from the defect outward and instructing the patient to report when the color improves or appears.

Automated Perimetry

Automated perimetry had its initial role in the early diagnosis and management of glaucoma patients. Although testing strategies are different, the use of automated perimetry in pathway disease of neuro-ophthalmic significance has gained increasing popularity, making it the test of choice for nearly all visual field defects. Automated techniques involve static testing using suprathreshold, threshold, and threshold-related strategies. The suprathreshold and threshold-related strategies are used in various screening programs involving central and peripheral portions of the field. Threshold strategies are extremely sensitive, repeatable, and accurate; however, they have the disadvantage of being time-consuming and therefore much more difficult for the patient to perform.[10] For threshold visual fields to be cost-effective and provide meaningful data, they are usually limited to smaller and typically central portions of the visual field.

Visual pathway disease has a predilection for the central visual fields; therefore, automated static perimetry emphasizing the central 24 or 30 degrees is the test of choice when visual field testing is recommended. Like glaucomatous disease, nonglaucomatous optic nerve disease has a predilection for the central 30 degrees. Further back in the visual pathway, diseases located at the chiasm and posterior produce hemianopic visual field defects, and although such defects will often extend to the periphery, they also have a predilection for the central field. Therefore, in most situations, central 24- or 30-degree threshold programs in which test points offset the vertical and horizontal hemianopic lines are ideal in neuro-ophthalmic disease. Although the preference varies from clinician to clinician, any model is appropriate if it has these capabilities. If the examiner wishes to obtain information beyond the central field, peripheral testing can be added to further qualify the extent of the defect. To save time, it is certainly appropriate to use suprathreshold or screening peripheral strategies in conjunction with central threshold strategies, particularly if qualitation of peripheral extension is all that is desired, and the defects are dense enough to ensure detection.

The great technologic strides made in automated perimetry have unfortunately made evaluation of defects more complicated. In manual types of perimetry, the examiner is able to ignore inconsistent or ambiguous responses and records only those that appear reliable. The result is clean visual field charts that are easily evaluated by the clinician. Although automated perimetry has the advantage of relieving the perimetrist of much of the work, it does not have the ability to ignore an invalid response. The result is an often messy-looking printout with defects hidden within a noisy background. This problem is perhaps more pronounced in neurologic patients who may be physically or mentally impaired and, hence, more apt to make mistakes. With these considerations in mind, it is especially crucial in neuro-ophthalmic disease to pay careful attention to the reliability indices that provide information on the validity of the field. These include false positives, false negatives, and fixation losses. It is important to understand that automation should never completely replace the perimetrist. For the test results to be valid, clear, simple instructions must be given to the patient. Careful monitoring throughout the test with coaching and encouragement as necessary are also prerequisites for obtaining useful studies. If it becomes clear during the early part of the test that the patient simply cannot perform, the test should be terminated to avoid unnecessary stress or frustration for the patient. Manual techniques should be used under such circumstances.

When examining the visual field printout, the examiner should look for defects consistent with neuro-ophthalmic disease. Optic nerve disease can cause central scotomas, arcuate defects, altitudinal defects, or generalized depressions. Generalized depressions from optic nerve disease will often have superimposed focal defects that are difficult to see. The pattern deviation of the Humphrey STATPAC statistical package (Humphrey Instruments, Inc., San Leandro, CA) will isolate focal depressions that are hidden within generalized depressions of all types, making them readily apparent to the examiner (Figure 3.5).

Because disease of the chiasm and posterior results in hemianopic defects, the examiner should pay special attention to the numeric threshold values on either side of the vertical hemianopic line, just as one does with the horizontal hemianopic line on the nasal side with glaucomatous visual field defects. Not only should the pairs of numbers immediately adjacent to the line be scrutinized, but corresponding pairs in the second and third columns should also be compared (Figure 3.6). If a vertical step

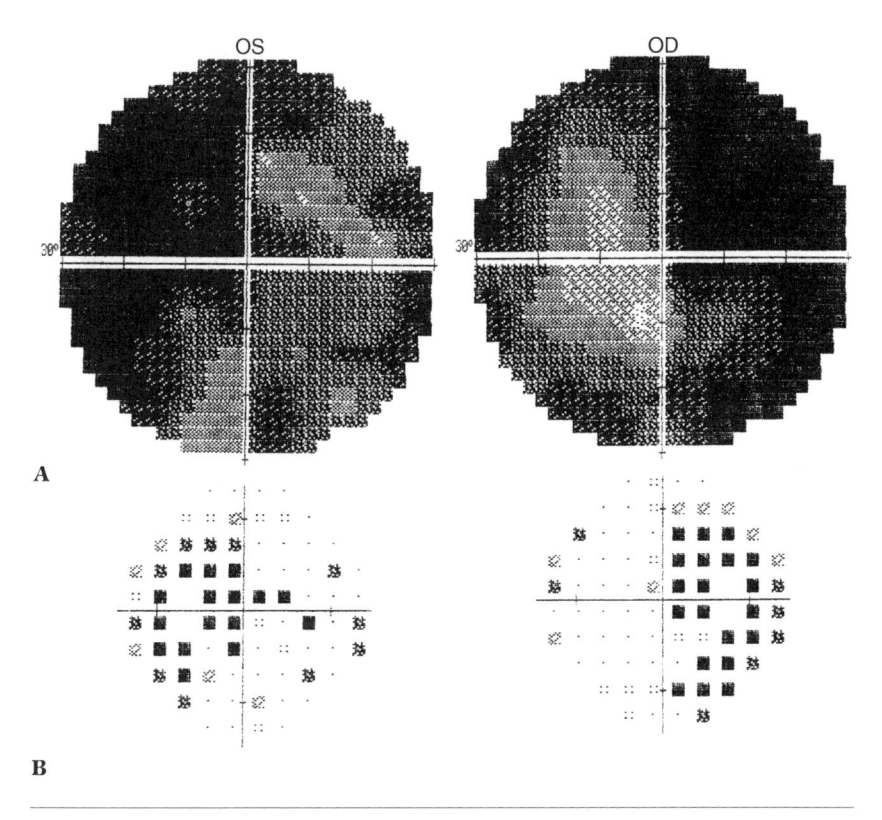

Figure 3.5 The gray scale (A) on this visual field appears to show overall depression, but the pattern deviation (B) of Humphrey's STATPAC statistical package will isolate focal depressions that are hidden within generalized depressions. Note how the pattern deviation reveals the bitemporal nature of the defect.

is present, the other eye should be carefully scrutinized. In disease of the chiasm and beyond, visual field defects will be bilateral (although early compression of the chiasm may be unilateral). Central screening tests are not as sensitive as their threshold counterparts; however, they have been shown to be nearly as effective in the detection of neuro-ophthalmic visual field defects.[11] Although confrontation testing using colored targets is believed by many to be equally sensitive to screening visual fields,[12,13] the former provides better documentation from a clinicolegal standpoint.

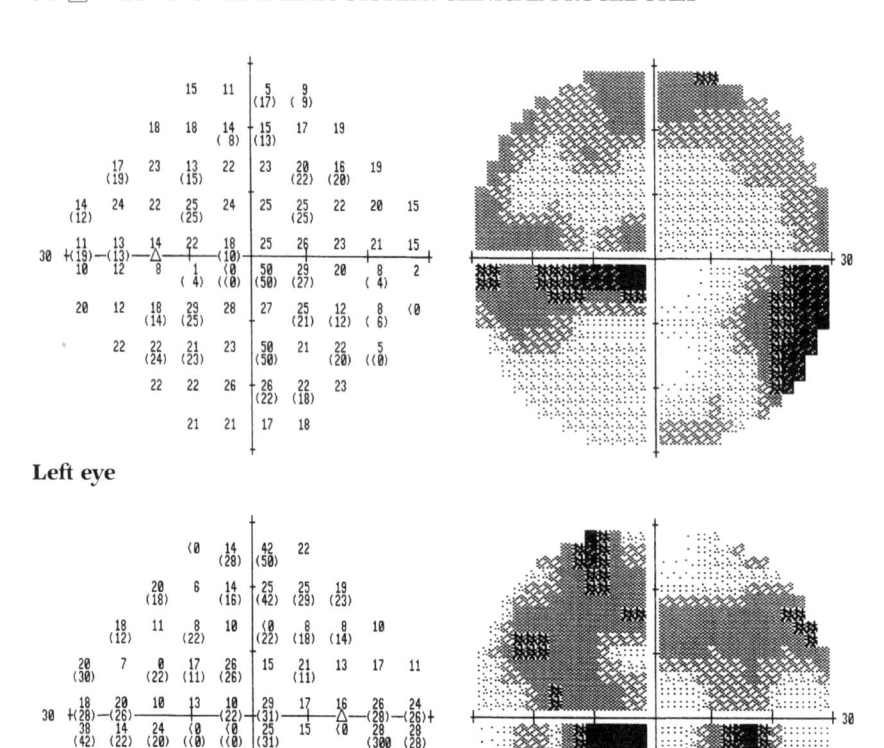

Figure 3.6 The left homonymous nature of field loss in this patient is not obvious, particularly in the right eye. Comparing corresponding rows of numbers on either side of the hemianopic line helps detect relative hemianopic loss.

Visual Field Defects in Nonglaucomatous Optic Nerve Disease

Visual field defects in optic nerve disease are unilateral except in cases in which there is a bilateral disease process. Often, there is an overall depres-

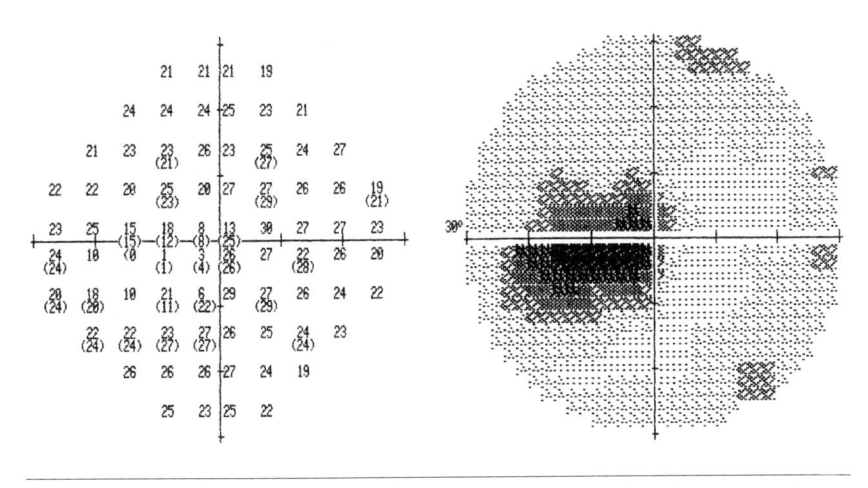

Figure 3.7 Cecocentral scotoma in the left eye of a patient with nutritional neuropathy. Note that the defect extends from the blind spot to fixation.

sion with superimposed focal deficits. This pattern of visual field loss is readily apparent on automated static threshold testing, but on Goldmann, overall depression is characterized by a constriction of isopters with superimposed focal defects. Other signs of optic nerve dysfunction are typically apparent and include reduced vision, color vision loss, and an afferent pupillary defect. Disc edema or pallor of the neuro-retinal rim are also important localizing features. One important rule of thumb in evaluating visual field defects in optic nerve disease is that patterns of neuro-retinal rim pallor correlate with patterns of visual field loss. Some common optic neuropathies and their visual field patterns follow.

■ Toxic and Nutritional Neuropathies

The optic neuropathy of chronic alcohol use, tobacco use, or both is characterized by gradual, symmetric, and painless vision loss with reduced color vision and cecocentral scotomas (Figure 3.7). Vision loss is typically in the range of 20/50 to 20/200 and is usually accompanied by temporal pallor of both optic nerves corresponding to the papillomacular bundles (Color Plate 5). This clinical profile mimics the optic neuropathy seen in severe malnutrition.[14] Thiamine,[15] folate,[16] and vitamin B_{12},[17,18] have all been implicated in tobacco/alcohol and nutritional optic neuropathies. Toxic neuropathies result in painless symmetric and bilateral vision loss, which may be abrupt or gradual. Vision loss is usually not severe but may be reduced beyond 20/200. The agents capable of producing toxic optic neuropathy are vast.[19]

The perimetric method of choice in approaching patients with toxic and nutritional neuropathies is automated perimetry with central threshold programs that include the blind spot. Because vision typically does not exceed 20/200, fixation is usually not a problem in automated testing. If the visual impairment is mild, the visual field defects may not be obvious on automated or Goldmann perimetry. Tangent screen fields using red targets may be helpful in such patients. The cecocentral scotomas are elicited by having the patients report changes in color saturation as a target is moved from fixation outward.

■ Optic Neuritis

Optic neuritis is characterized by an acute or subacute loss of vision in one eye with pain on eye movement. The optic nerve appearance is normal in most, with approximately one-third of patients demonstrating swelling (Color Plate 6). The visual field defects are varied and numerous.[20] Approximately half of patients with optic neuritis have diffuse defects, and the rest show localized defects. Of those with localized defects, altitudinal field loss is most common followed by patients with three quadrant visual loss and one quadrant visual field loss, respectively. Central and cecocentral scotomas are each seen with a frequency of only 4%.[20] Visual field defects in optic neuritis typically improve within 2 weeks, although residual defects will persist. In addition, subtle defects are often apparent in the fellow eyes and become more prevalent with time. Visual fields are best evaluated with threshold, central 30-degree programs on automated perimetry. This is far superior to manual approaches because overall depressions will show up better and because residual and fellow eye defects are typically subtle and very focal, making them easily overlooked with manual testing or automated screening programs. Visual fields should be evaluated in both eyes and should be repeated with each follow-up until vision returns. Even with the return of vision, new and different patterns of defects have been seen over the first-year follow-up period.[21]

■ Anterior Ischemic Optic Neuropathy

Anterior ischemic optic neuropathy is the result of hypoperfusion of the anterior portion of the optic nerve.[22] The result is infarction of the optic nerve with sudden loss of vision, disc edema (Color Plate 7), an afferent pupillary defect, and visual field loss. Characteristic visual field defects include altitudinal defects, arcuate defects, quadrant defects, and central scotomas, in that order of frequency,[23] with the arteritic form exhibiting more severe visual field loss than the nonarteritic form.[23,24] In most cases, the visual field defects can be documented with central threshold programs. If the patient finds this difficult, Goldmann perimetry is the next option (Figure 3.8). Fields should be monitored at regular intervals for the first 4 weeks. The majority of patients will remain stable or recover a line or two of Snellen acuity, whereas others will progress in a stuttering fashion in the initial weeks.[25]

■ Pseudotumor Cerebri

Pseudotumor cerebri (PTC) (Color Plate 8), or benign intracranial hypertension, is a disorder that most commonly affects obese women of childbearing age.[26] Although it is typically referred to as a benign disorder, the chronic papilledema that results from increased intracranial pressure can result in axonal damage and visual field loss. Visual field loss in PTC is typically gradual and often asymptomatic in the early stages. Although enlarged blind spots are the earliest and most common visual field defect seen in PTC, they are due to the edema itself rather than nerve fiber loss and disappear with resolution of the edema. Persistence of papilledema results in nerve fiber loss–associated visual field defects, which include overall depression, inferonasal loss, paracentral defects, arcuate scotomas, temporal wedge defects, and altitudinal loss.[27] Visual field loss is best demonstrated with automated central threshold programs, with defects seen in nearly 70%.[26] Severe defects are seen in approximately 10% (Figure 3.9).[25,26] Despite resolution of papilledema, increased cerebrospinal fluid pressure is often persistent, and there is a 10% recurrence rate.[28] Therefore, patients should undergo threshold visual field testing initially as a baseline and monthly for the first 3 months. Testing should

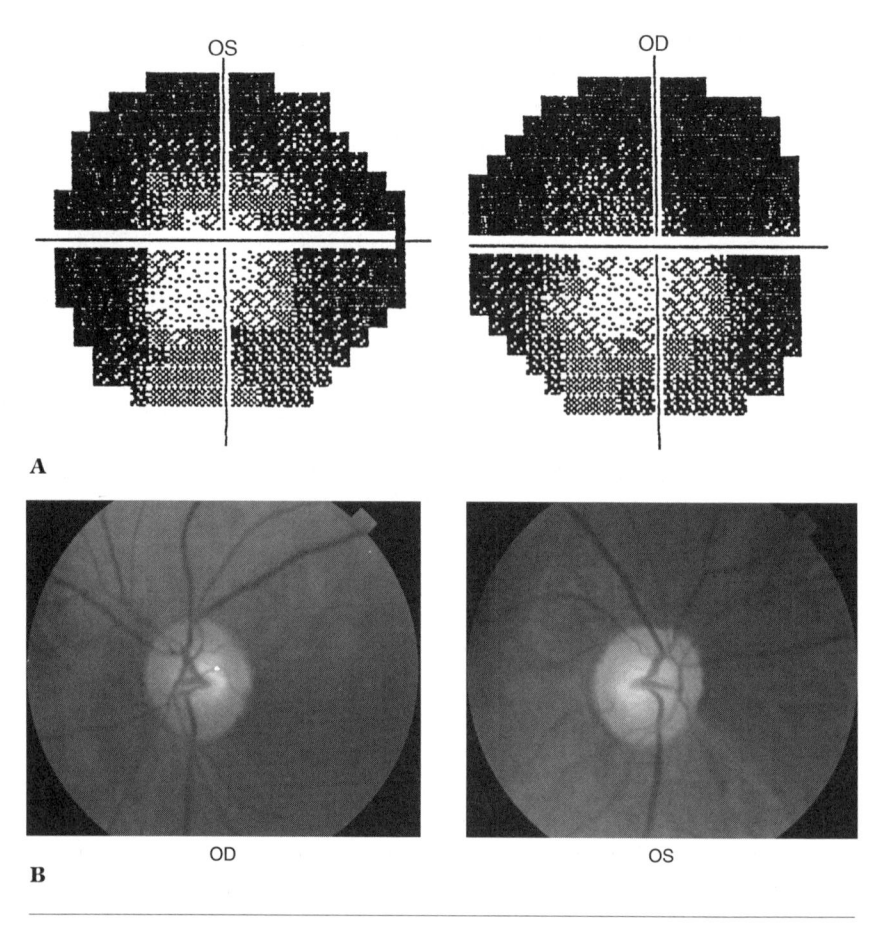

Figure 3.8 This patient with an old, mild ischemic optic neuropathy did not perform well on automated threshold testing (A). The extent of visual field loss does not correlate with the optic nerve appearance (B). Manual perimetry does a much better job of qualifying her visual field loss (C,D).

then be repeated every 3–4 months as long as the disc edema persists. The duration of the disease ranges from 1–28 months; however, the recurrence rate is 12% and disease may occur years later.[27] Therefore, patients should have yearly follow-up with repeat visual fields after presumed resolution of the condition.

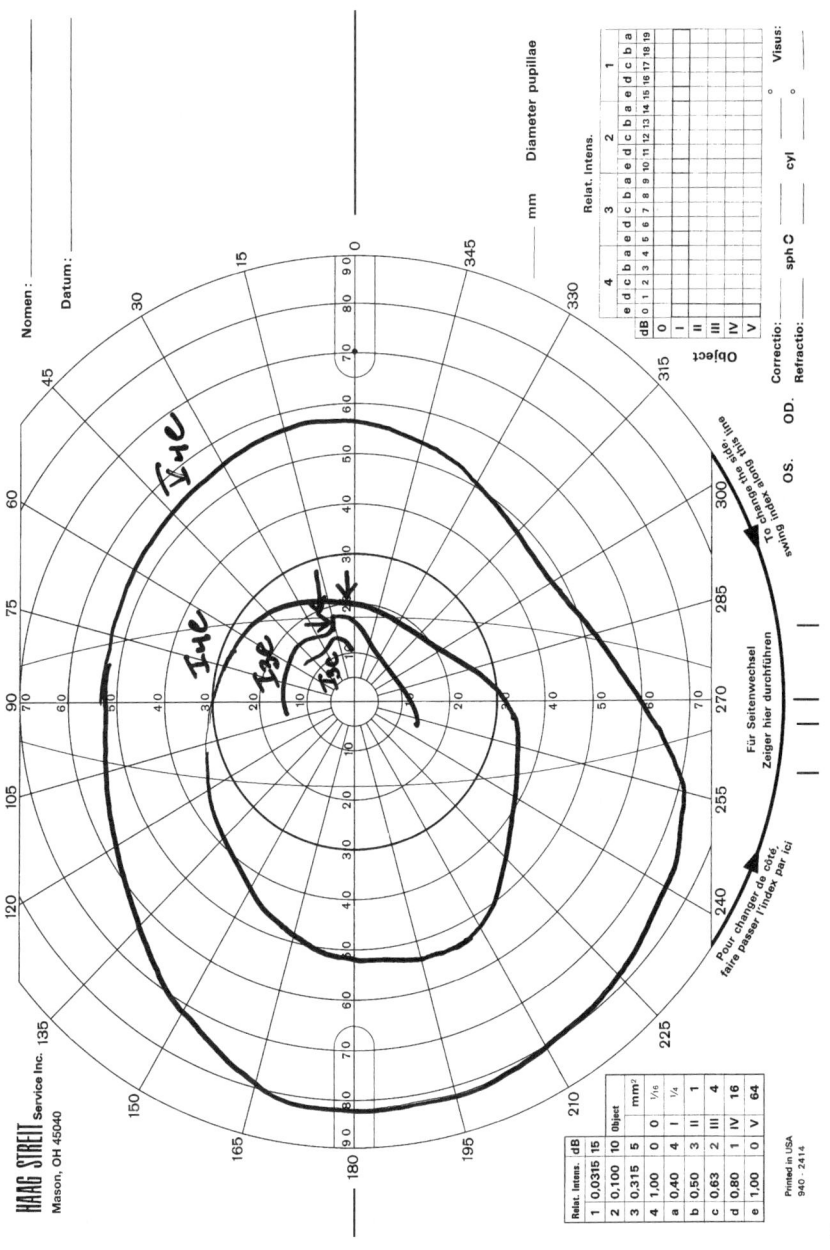

Visual Field Evaluation in Neuro-Ophthalmic Disease □ 89

NEURO-OPHTHALMIC SYSTEM: CLINICAL PROCEDURES

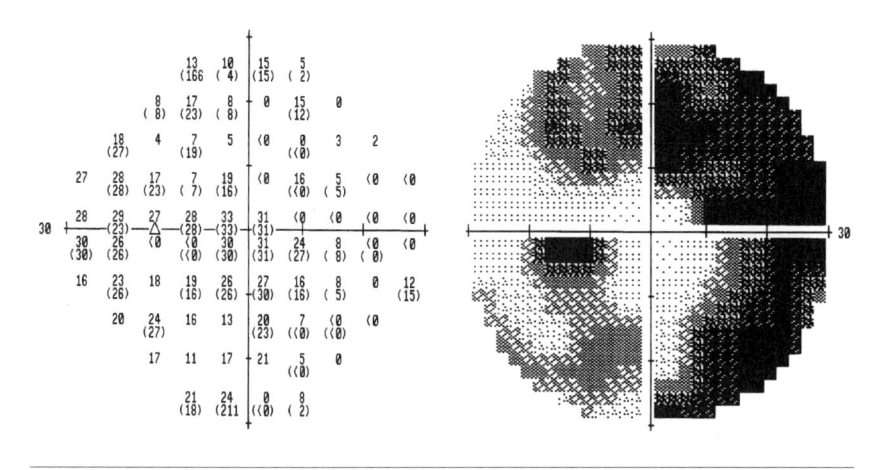

Figure 3.9 Extensive visual field loss in the left eye of a patient with chronic atrophic papilledema.

■ Congenital Optic Nerve Anomalies

Congenital anomalies of the optic nerves mimic optic nerve disease processes not only by their appearance, but also by the visual field defects they produce. Pseudopapilledema from a congenitally anomalous optic nerve must be distinguished from true papilledema or other pathologic processes causing disc edema because the former does not require the inconvenience and expense of an extensive medical workup. The congenitally anomalous disc is a small, elevated nerve without a physiologic cup. The elevation is the result of crowded axons within a small scleral canal. This pseudopapilledema can be distinguished from true disc edema by the appearance of the peripapillary vasculature. In true optic nerve head edema, nerve fiber layer swelling results in obscuration and congestion of the peripapillary vasculature, whereas in pseudopapilledema, the disc vasculature remains clear through the elevated

◄ **Figure 3.8** (D) *Continued.*

disc tissue, and there is no evidence of vascular compromise. The vascular pattern seen in congenitally anomalous discs will often show unusual branching patterns consisting of multiple trifurcations and quadrifurcations. Optic nerve drusen, or hyalin bodies, are often seen with careful ophthalmoscopy as bright, yellowish areas that give the disc a lumpy appearance with scalloped margins (Color Plate 9). Often, the drusen are buried too deeply to be visualized ophthalmoscopically, but associated calcific changes make them easily visible with B-scan ultrasound. Visual field defects are seen in many patients with disc drusen, and these mimic the enlarged blind spots and arcuate defects seen in chronic papilledema.[29] Further complicating the differential diagnosis is the fact that visual field defects associated with disc drusen are progressive and often result in significant visual field constriction, although central acuity is rarely affected. Although there is no treatment for optic nerve drusen, patients should undergo regular visual field testing, preferably with central, threshold programs, because the visual field loss is progressive and often significant.

Optic nerve hypoplasia occurs when there is a subnormal number of axons in the optic nerve. The spectrum ranges from mild to severe, the former often escaping diagnosis. Ophthalmoscopically, the disc is smaller than normal and, in more obvious cases, is surrounded by a peripapillary halo (Color Plate 10). The outer ring of the halo represents the junction between the sclera and lamina cribrosa, and the inner ring is the termination of the retinal pigment epithelium.[30] Because hypoplastic nerves have a reduced number of axons, reduced acuity and visual field defects are common. These include arcuate, altitudinal, or temporal depressions.[31] Defects can be documented with automated or manual techniques and should remain stable over time.

Optic nerve colobomas are excavations of the disc that may extend into the retina and choroid. The excavation of optic nerve colobomas can sometimes mimic glaucomatous cupping (Color Plate 11) with the distinction that the ophthalmoscopic appearance and associated visual field defects do not show progression. Optic pits are small, incomplete colobomas that usually occur on the inferotemporal aspect of the disc (Color Plate 12). Arcuate visual field defects are typically seen with optic pits, and these, too, remain unchanged over time.

Tilted discs occur when there is an oblique insertion of the optic nerve into the globe. The disc has an oval shape with an associated crescent (Color Plate 13). Visual field loss is common, and often patients have bitemporal depressions. These can be distinguished from the bitemporal visual field loss of chiasmal compression, because they cross over the vertical hemianopic line and extend into the nasal field. As with most other congenital anomalies, the visual field defects remain stable over time. Often, tilted discs are seen in conjunction with oblique myopic astigmatism.

Visual Field Defects in Chiasmal Disease

The classic visual field defects seen in disease of the chiasm are the result of its anatomic relationship to the sella turcica, which houses the pituitary gland. Bitemporal hemianopia is the hallmark of chiasmal compression from an enlarging pituitary adenoma, which is the most common etiology of the "chiasmal syndrome."[32] Tumors of the pituitary gland impinge on the chiasm from below, compressing the crossed, medially located, inferior nasal fibers that represent temporal visual field. As the mass enlarges, the visual field defect enlarges to involve the inferior temporal field. If the mass encroaches on the temporal aspect of the chiasm, the nasal field eventually becomes involved, beginning inferiorly. Although this is the classically described pattern of visual field loss, the actual clinical presentation of visual field defects from chiasmal compression due to pituitary adenoma depends on the location of the chiasm with respect to the sella turcica. Depending on the position of the chiasm with respect to the sella turcica, pituitary tumors may compress the optic nerves or optic tracts, resulting in central scotoma or homonymous hemianopia in isolation or in conjunction with bitemporal visual field loss (Figure 3.10). Disease of the chiasm also includes compres-

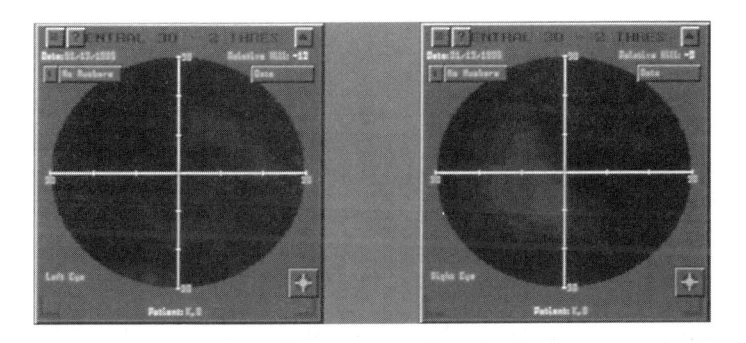

Figure 3.10 Dicon (Dicon Inc., San Diego, CA) threshold 30-degree program visual field showing extensive visual field loss in a patient with a large pituitary adenoma. In addition to bitemporal involvement, there is central involvement.

sion from other tumors (e.g., craniopharyngiomas, gliomas, meningiomas), vascular disease, inflammation, infection, aneurysm, and trauma. The visual field defects in these disorders are less predictable and depend on the particular fibers of the chiasm that are affected.

Visual field analysis using automated, threshold approaches has been shown to be more effective, sensitive, and reproducible compared with manual Goldmann techniques in the detection of even minimal defects due to chiasmal disease.[33,34] Goldmann techniques can be used as a second option, and sensitivity can be improved by paying careful attention to the central 30 degrees.[35] Visual fields should be well documented before referring the patient for surgical and/or medical management of the underlying condition. Fields should be repeated as early as possible after treatment begins and monitored at regular intervals (Figure 3.11). In most cases of sellar or chiasmal neoplasms, the possibility of recurrence always exists; therefore, once fields stabilize, they should be repeated at 6- to 12-month intervals to rule out further progression.

Postchiasmal Pathway Disease

Before discussion of visual field defects produced by postchiasmal pathway disease, the reader must be familiar with several concepts regarding the visual field defects produced by postchiasmal disease. Diseases of the optic tracts and posterior produce visual field defects that are homonymous—that is, they involve the nasal field of one eye and the temporal field of the fellow eye. In addition, defects are characterized by congruity. Defects that are congruous are those in which the nasal and temporal defects closely resemble one another, whereas those that are incongruous do not. In general, after the pathway fibers cross in the chiasm and course posteriorly, they become increasingly segregated with regard to the areas of the visual field they represent. Therefore, a general rule of thumb is that the more posterior in the visual pathway the lesion, the more congruous the visual field defect produced by the lesion becomes. There are some exceptions to this rule. Decreased visual acuity does not occur in postchiasmal disease unless the lesion simultaneously involves both the right and left sides of the visual pathway, as is often the case in disease of the occipital lobes.

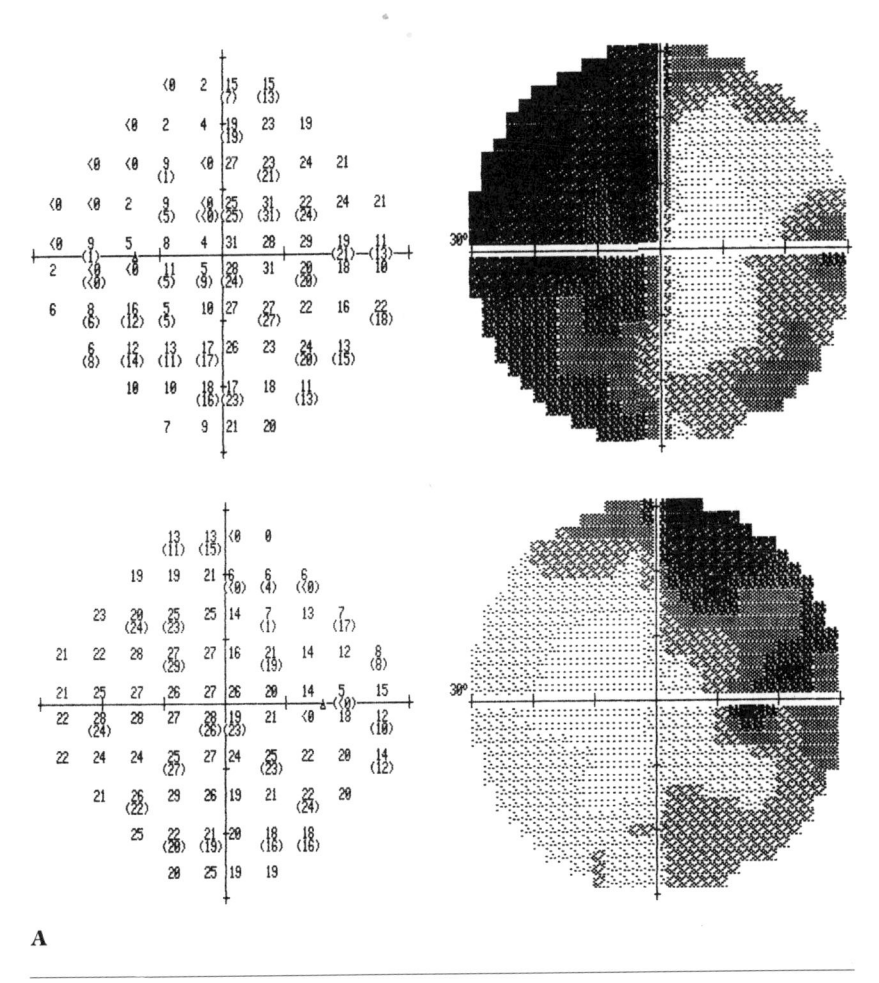

Figure 3.11 (A) Central 30-2 visual fields showing bitemporal visual field loss in the left eye (top) and right eye (bottom) in a patient with a pituitary adenoma.

■ Optic Tract Disease

Isolated lesions of the optic tract are rare[36] and typically result in incongruous homonymous hemianopias. Often, the offending lesions are compressive and involve the chiasm and ipsilateral optic nerve to produce signs of chiasmal and optic nerve disease in addition to homony-

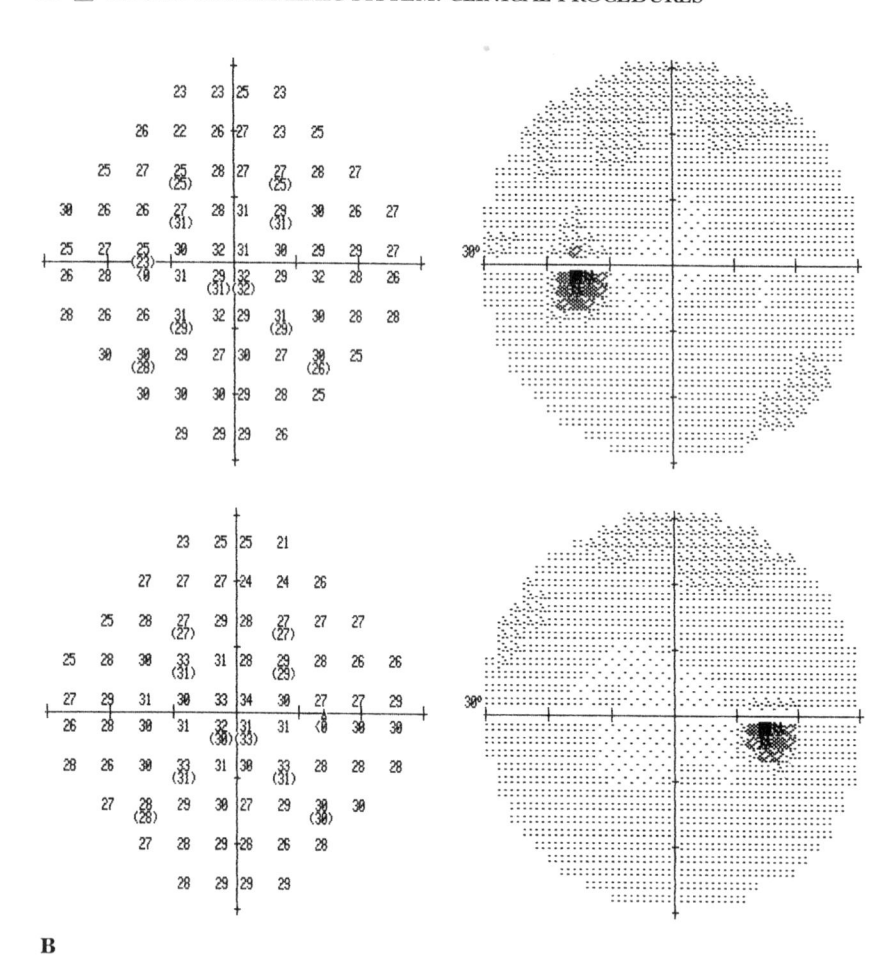

```
              23  23 |25  23
           26  22  26|27  23  25
       25  27  25  28|27  27  28  27
              (25)       (25)
    30 26  26  27  28|31  29  30  26  27
              (31)       (31)
    25  27  25  30  32|31  30  29  29  27
   ─26──28──(23)──31──29─32──29──32──28──26─
                     (31)(32)
    28  26  26  31  32|29  31  30  28  28
              (29)       (29)
       30  30  29  27|30  27  30  25
          (28)             (26)
           30  30  30|29  28  25
              29  29 |29  26
```

```
              23  25 |25  21
           27  27  27|24  24  26
       25  28  27  29|28  27  27  27
              (27)       (27)
    25  28  30  33  31|28  29  28  26  26
              (31)       (29)
    27  29  31  30  33|34  30  27  27  29
   ─26──28──30──31──32─31──31──(0─30──30─
                     (30)(33)
    28  26  30  33  31|30  33  28  28  28
              (31)       (31)
       27  28  29  30|27  29  30  30
          (28)             (30)
           27  28  29|28  26  28
              28  29 |29  29
```

B

Figure 3.11 *Continued.* After surgery to remove a pituitary adenoma, the field returns to normal (B).

mous hemianopia. When lesions are truly isolated to the tracts, however, some important associations with the visual field defects exist. There is typically an afferent pupillary defect in the contralateral eye[37] (with the temporal visual field loss) and a band pattern of optic atrophy in the contralateral eye (Color Plate 14). Invasion of the nearby diencephalon may also result in endocrine dysfunction due to hypothalamic involvement.[38]

■ Lateral Geniculate Body

Visual pathway fibers synapse in the lateral geniculate nucleus (LGN) before continuing their posterior course in the optic radiations. The visual field defects in LGN disease are of two basic types: The first is a homonymous horizontal sectoranopia[39]; the second is a loss of upper and lower homonymous sectors of field.[40] The unique characteristics of these visual fields are best visualized with visual field programs that include the periphery. Automated, full-field threshold programs provide the best information; however, the length of time required to perform these tests makes them less appealing and difficult for the patient. Therefore, Goldmann visual fields are ideal. If Goldmann is not available, full-field screening programs are useful. Screening strategies such as the "three-zone" and "quantify defects" options of the Humphrey perimeter provide additional information regarding missed points. Although additional test time is needed with these programs, they are still faster than full-field threshold techniques. Despite being located in the anterior portion of the visual field, the defects seen in LGN disease are usually congruous.

■ Temporal Lobe

The visual field defects that result from temporal lobe lesions are typically incongruous, pie-shaped, homonymous hemianopias that are denser above the horizontal raphe with sloping inferior margins. The defects are congruous or incongruous and do not spare the peripheral field. Vascular lesions in the temporal lobe are less common causes of temporal lobe disease, with tumors and abscesses predominating.[41] Patients with visual field defects from temporal lobe disease rarely present to the optometrist because their accompanying neurologic signs and symptoms overshadow their visual symptoms. Seizures are common and may be preceded by an unpleasant odor or taste. Auditory or visual hallucinations occur as well. The associated neurologic impairments often make it difficult to obtain formal visual fields. If formal documentation of visual fields is desired, manual perimetric techniques are often indicated. These allow prompt visualization of both the central and peripheral visual fields.

Parietal Lobe

Homonymous hemianopias from parietal lobe disease are typically congruous. Because the optic radiations course completely within the parietal lobe, the visual field defects can involve both the superior and inferior portions of the field (Figure 3.12). In addition to the visual field defects, parietal lobe lesions have other important ocular features. Spasticity of conjugate gaze[42] is a tonic deviation of the eyes to the side opposite the lesion when attempting to produce a Bell's reflex (upward deviation of the eyes on forced eyelid closure). Asymmetry of optokinetic nystagmus[38] is also an important feature. On passing an optokinetic stimulus toward the side of the lesion, the response is diminished or absent, whereas passing the stimulus toward the normal side produces normal optokinetic eye movements.

In extensive parietal lobe disease, the visual field defects are often overshadowed by neurologic signs and symptoms. Such patients are less likely to present initially to an optometrist and are more frequently seen in inpatient neurologic settings. Due to the nature of neurologic associations, visual field defects in extensive parietal lobe disease are often difficult, if not impossible, to formally record. Furthermore, patients with parietal lobe disease are often unaware of their defects, further complicating diagnosis.

Occipital Lobe

In the occipital lobe, visual pathway fibers become so segregated that precise congruity is the rule (Figure 3.13). Because the occipital lobes are divided into superior and inferior lips, quadrantic defects are frequently seen. Also, because both halves of the visual pathway are now in close proximity and share a common blood supply, it is possible for a single lesion to involve both halves of the visual field simultaneously (Figure 3.14).

Figure 3.12 ▶ Incongruous left homonymous hemianopia from a right parietal lobe lesion. The central 30-2 and peripheral 60-2 programs of the Humphrey automated perimeter have been merged to show the whole extent of the defect.

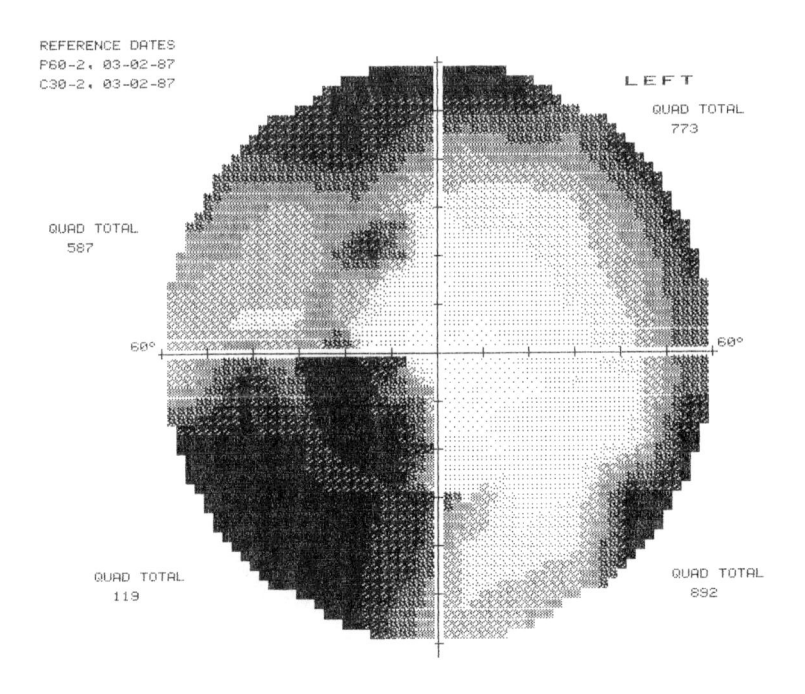

Visual Field Evaluation in Neuro-Ophthalmic Disease □ **99**

REFERENCE DATES
P60-2, 03-02-87
C30-2, 03-02-87

LEFT
QUAD TOTAL
773

QUAD TOTAL
587

60°   60°

QUAD TOTAL
119

QUAD TOTAL
892

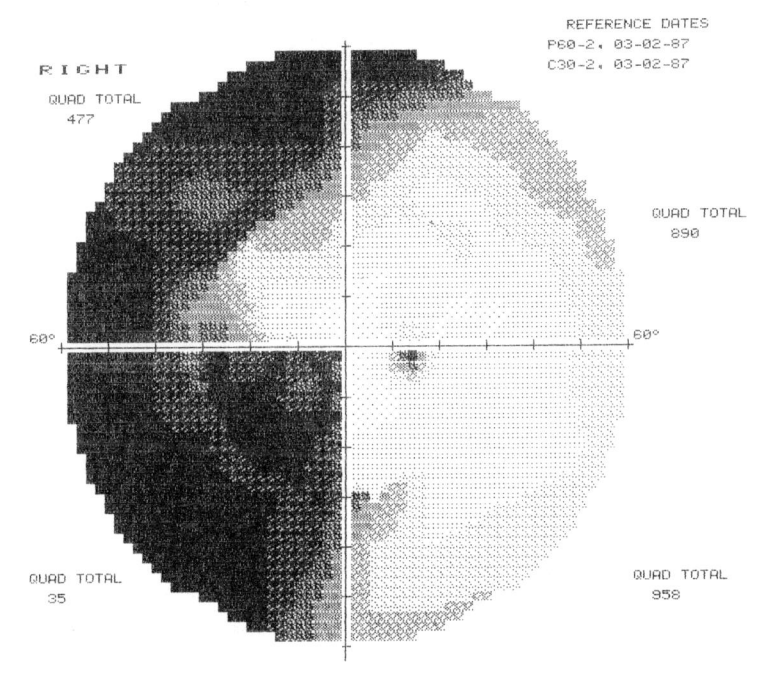

REFERENCE DATES
P60-2, 03-02-87
C30-2, 03-02-87

RIGHT
QUAD TOTAL
477

QUAD TOTAL
890

60°   60°

QUAD TOTAL
35

QUAD TOTAL
958

Left eye

Right eye

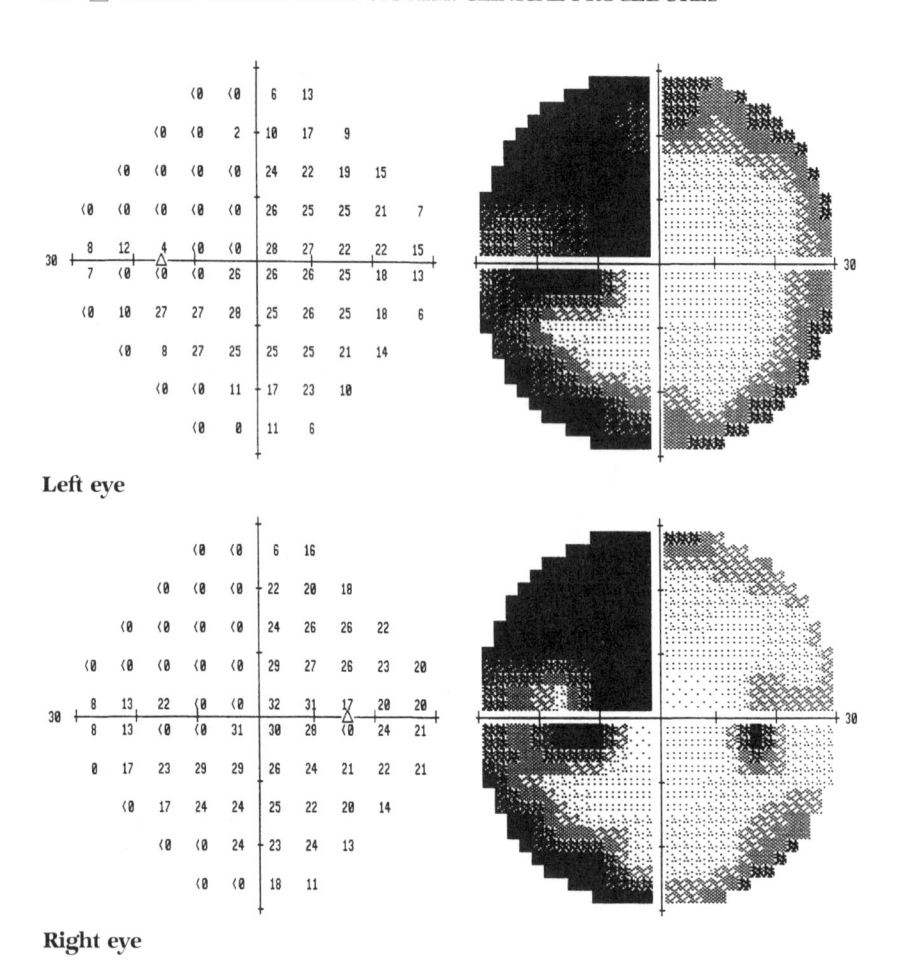

Figure 3.13 Precise congruity is demonstrated in this left homonymous hemianopia from a right occipital lobe infarction.

Two unique characteristics are seen in the visual fields in occipital lobe disease. The first is macular sparing. To this point, postchiasmal visual field defects will typically split fixation—that is, they respect the vertical meridian through fixation. In occipital lobe disease, however, it is possible that the central 10 degrees or less of visual field on the involved side will be preserved (Figure 3.15). Clinical evidence shows that this occurs when the occipital lobe tip is spared in occipital lobe disease.[43]

Left eye

Right eye

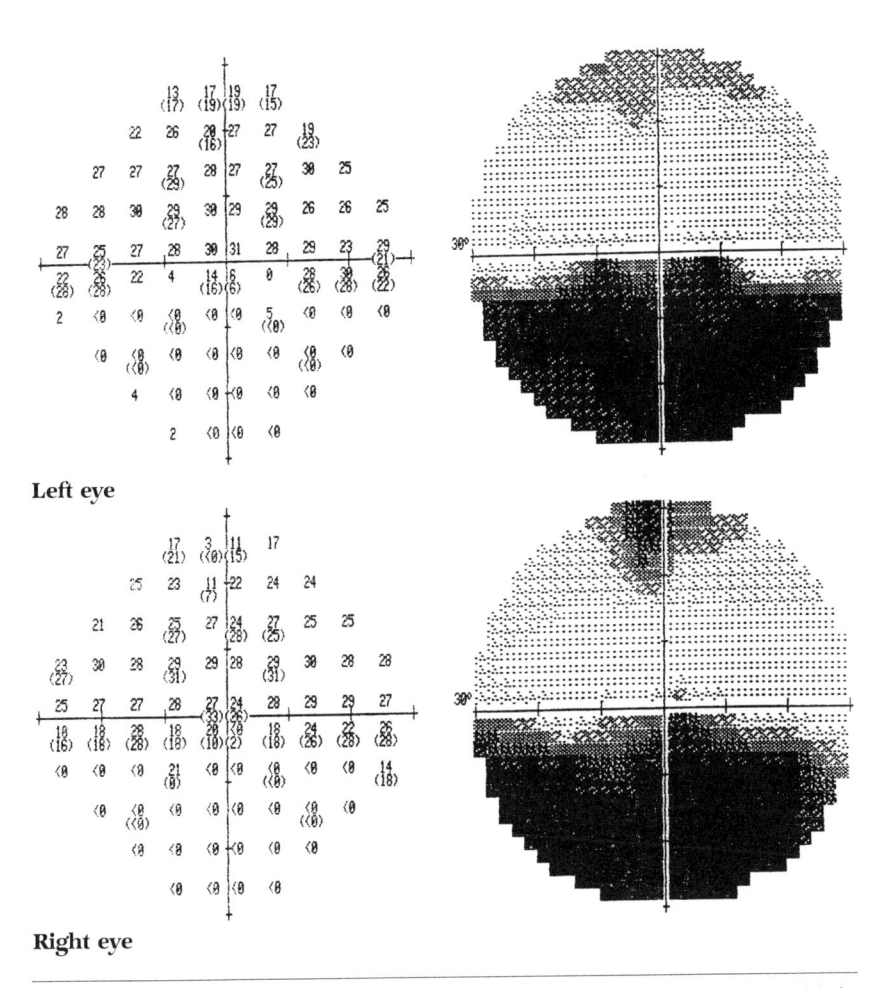

Figure 3.14 A lesion in the superior occipital lobe involving the right and left halves results in a visual field defect that involves the left and right halves of the inferior visual field.

A dual blood supply to the occipital lobe has been hypothesized to explain this occurrence.[44] The second unique characteristic of occipital lobe disease is that of preservation of the temporal crescent. The anterior region of the occipital lobe adjacent to the interhemispheric fissure

Figure 3.15 ▶ Macular sparing in occipital lobe disease demonstrated by Goldmann perimetry. (A) Left eye. (B) Right eye.

102 □ NEURO-OPHTHALMIC SYSTEM: CLINICAL PROCEDURES

B

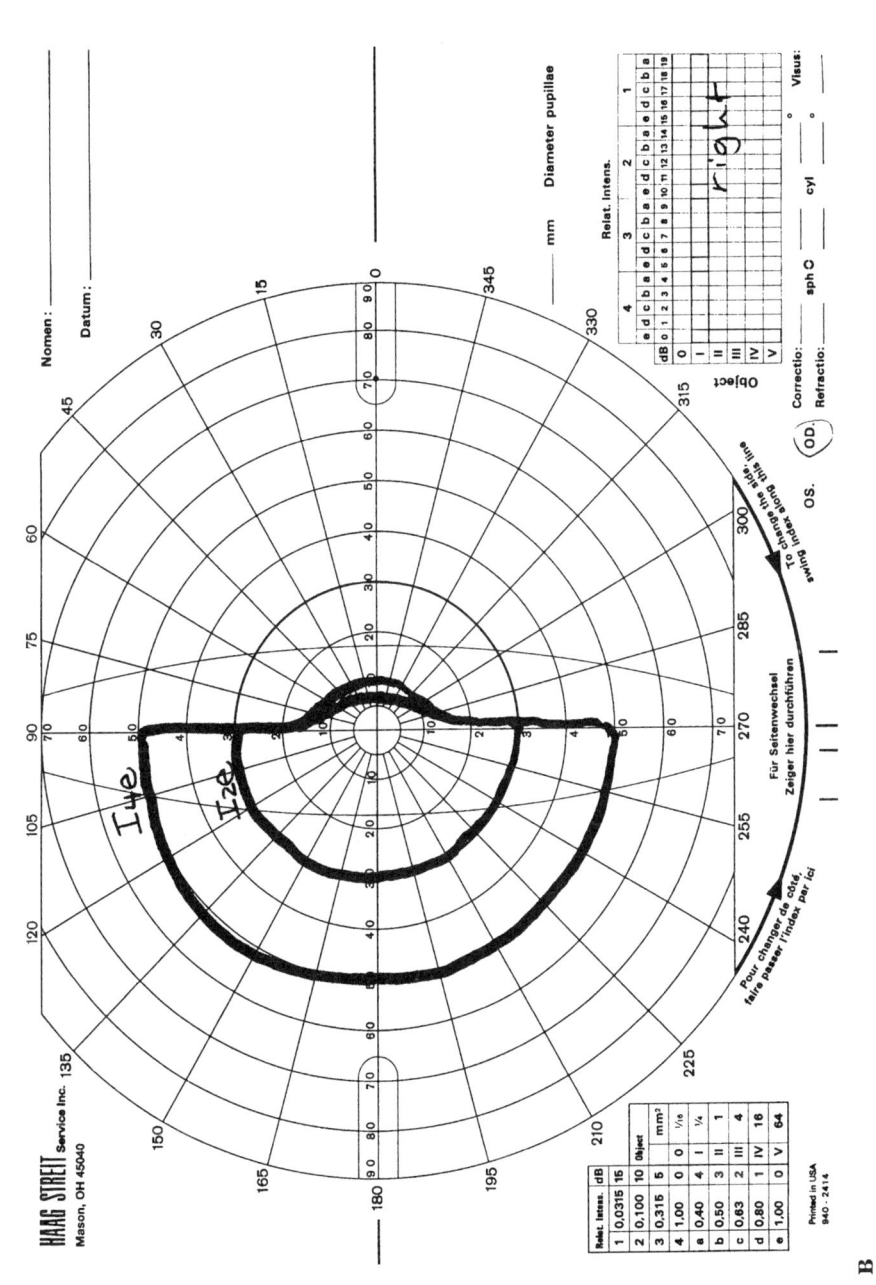

receives unilateral input from the contralateral temporal field. Therefore, when this area is spared in occipital lobe strokes, there is an intact peripheral temporal field contralateral to the lesion.

Visual field defects from occipital lobe disease are perhaps the most common postchiasmal visual field defects seen in outpatient optometric settings. Often, patients are unaware of their defects, even when they result from ischemic disease, and it is not unusual to discover small, paracentral homonymous defects on routine testing. The defects seen in occipital lobe disease are typically the result of infarction. Isolated occipital lobe disease is not usually associated with neurologic signs. Documenting occipital visual field defects with formal perimetry is easily and best accomplished with threshold perimetry. Because the defects have a predilection for the central 30 degrees and many small, paracentral defects are completely confined within it, central 30-degree programs are ideal and often central 10-degree programs are quite useful (Figure 3.16). Patients with visual field defects should be monitored for improvement. A typical follow-up pattern includes repeat testing at 1 month, 3 months, 6 months, and then yearly.

Functional Visual Field Loss

Patients without organic visual pathway disease will often demonstrate visual field defects. These defects can be intentionally feigned as in malingering or may be unintentional, as is often seen in hysterical patients. Whatever the underlying nature of the disturbance, functional visual field loss has certain characteristics that differentiate it from true organic pathway disease. The functional patient will often report tunnel vision, which can be demonstrated with formal perimetry. Careful scrutiny of results will often reveal high numbers of false negatives on automated fields,

---

Figure 3.16 ▶   This patient has a small, paracentral, homonymous hemianopic defect. Note that the defect appears insignificant with a full-field screening program (A) but is much better qualified with a 10-2 threshold program (B).

LEFT

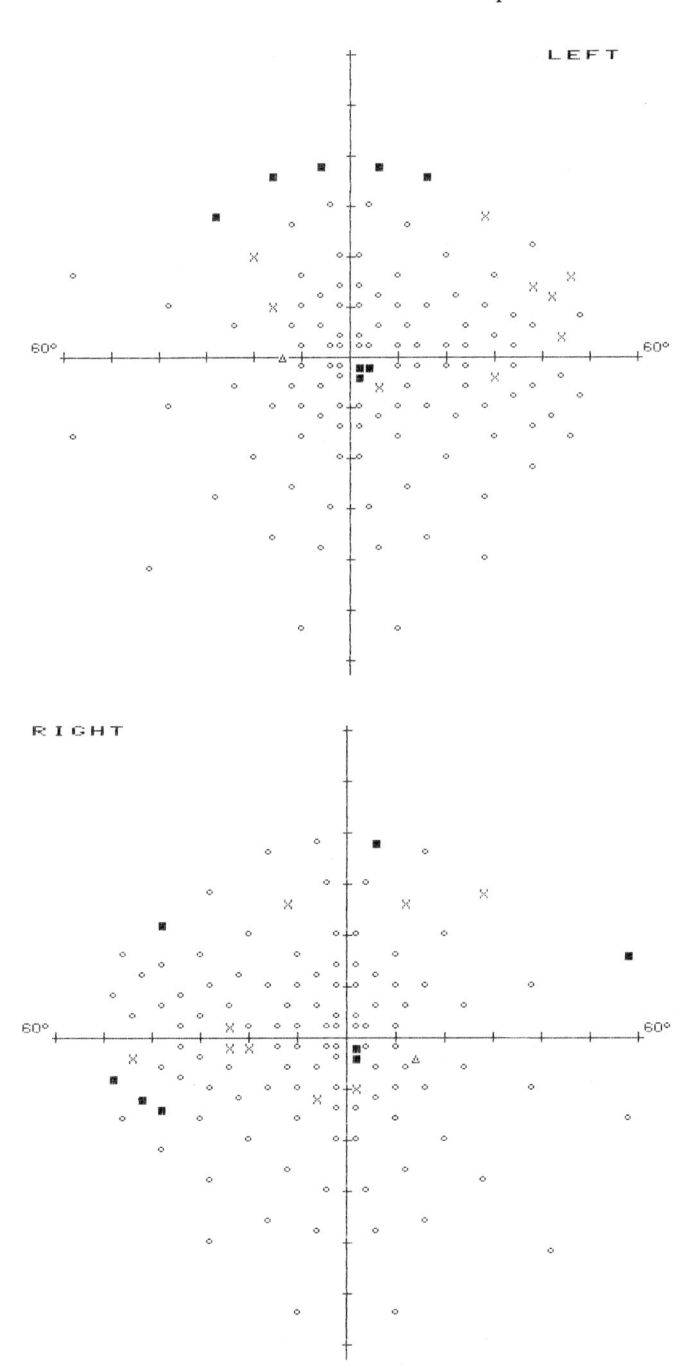

60°   60°

RIGHT

60°   60°

A

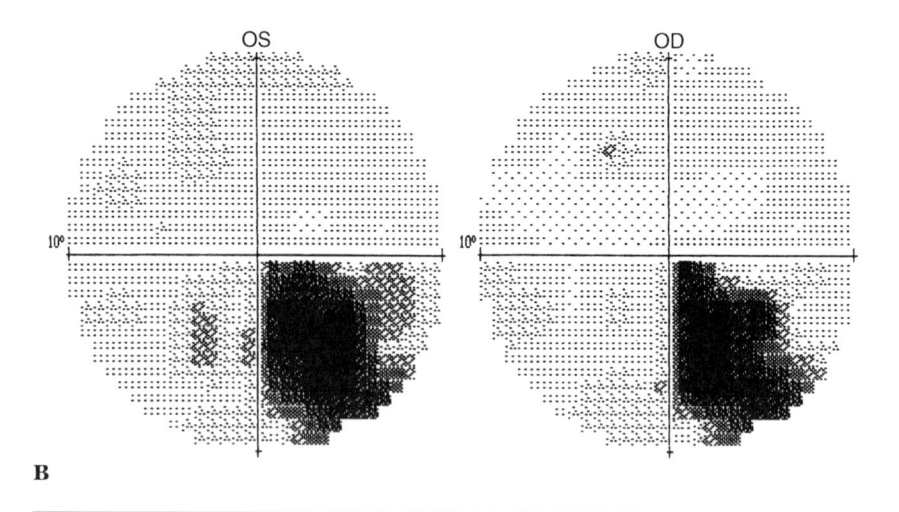

Figure 3.16 *Continued.*

with overlapped isopters and inconsistent responses on manual perimetry. Confrontation testing often shows severely constricted fields; however, patients who are feigning will often give themselves away by making a telltale saccade to a peripheral stimulus (the same may be noted when fixation is observed during formal perimetry). Despite severely compromised visual fields, these patients do not have the associated mobility limitations that are seen with true visual field compromise. The best way to document functionally constricted visual fields is by performing tangent screen testing at both 1-m and 2-m test distances, being sure to double the stimulus size at 2 m. Patients with functional visual field constriction will mistakenly believe that the visual field should constrict or remain the same when the test distance is doubled. In addition to tunnel vision, other types of visual field defects are also seen, particularly with malingerers. It is best not to investigate such defects with automated perimeters, however, because even patients with minimal knowledge of the visual pathways have been shown to possess the ability to reliably feign neurologic field loss on automated testing.[45] In such cases, careful clinical evaluation will detect inconsistencies among examination findings that suggest malingering. In addition, malingerers will often reveal financial motivations for their actions, such as impending litigation and disability benefits.

Billing and Reimbursement

Visual fields performed by confrontation are considered part of a comprehensive examination and therefore cannot be billed as a separate procedure. Tangent screen, Goldmann, and computerized visual field testing are billable as separate procedures. Codes exist for three levels of evaluation. Limited visual field (92081) is for a single stimulus level test such as a tangent screen or computerized screening strategy. Intermediate visual field (92082) is for testing at least two isopters on a Goldmann field or a computerized, suprathreshold screening strategy. Extended visual fields (92083) apply to at least three isopters of testing on Goldmann or computerized full-threshold perimetry.

Code	Goldmann	Automated	Approximate reimbursement
92081	1 isopter	Screening	$25–35
92082	2 isopters	Suprathreshold screening	$35–45
92083	3 or more isopters	Threshold	$45–55

■ Related International Classification of Diseases-9 (ICD-9) Terminology

Papilledema	377.01
Optic atrophy (primary)	377.11
Optic atrophy (postinflammatory)	377.12
Optic atrophy (partial)	377.15
Optic atrophy (hereditary)	377.16
Optic nerve drusen	377.21
Optic nerve coloboma	377.23
Pseudopapilledema	377.24
Optic neuritis	377.30
Papillitis	377.31
Nutritional optic neuropathy	377.33
Toxic optic neuropathy	377.34
Ischemic optic neuropathy	377.41
Optic nerve compression	377.49

Chiasmal syndrome	377.5
Associated with pituitary tumor	377.51
Associated with other neoplasm	377.52
Associated with vascular disease	377.53
Associated with inflammatory disease	377.54
Disorders of visual cortex	377.7
Associated with neoplasm	377.71
Associated with vascular disease	377.72
Associated with inflammation	377.73
Cortical blindness	377.75
Central/cecocentral scotoma	368.41
Arcuate scotoma	368.43
Homonymous hemianopia	368.46
Bitemporal/binasal hemianopia	368.47

■ References

1. Kirkham TH. The ocular symptomatology of pituitary tumors. Proc R Soc Med 1972;65:517–518.
2. Harrington DO, Drake MV. The Visual Fields—Text and Atlas of Clinical Perimetry. St. Louis: Mosby, 1990;1.
3. Edge K. The visual field in normal subjects. Acta Ophthalmol (Copenh) 1984;169(Suppl):1.
4. Traquair HM. An Introduction to Clinical Perimetry (6th ed). London: Kingston, 1949.
5. Bender MB, Furlow LT. Phenomenon of visual extinction in homonymous fields and the psychologic principles involved. Arch Neurol Psychiatr 1945;53:29.
6. Bender MB, Kanzer MG. Dynamics of homonymous hemianopsias and preservation of central vision. Brain 1939;62:404–421.
7. Johnson CA, Keltner JL. Optimal rates of movement for kinetic perimetry. Arch Ophthalmol 1987;105:73–75.
8. Riddoch G. Dissociation in visual perceptions due to occipita injuries, with especial references to appreciation of movement. Brain 1917;40:15–57.
9. Zappia RJ, Enoch JM, Stamper R, et al. The Riddoch phenomenon revealed in non-occipital lobe lesions. Br J Ophthalmol 1971;55:416–420.
10. Milder B. A.P.E. (acute perimeter exhaustion syndrome). Surv Ophthalmol 1987;32:148.
11. Siatkowski RM, Lam BL, Anderson DR, et al. Automated suprathreshold static perimetry screening for detecting neuro-ophthalmologic disease. Opthalmology 1996;103:907–917.

12. Frisen L. A versatile color confrontation test for the central visual field. A comparison with quantitative perimetry. Arch Opthalmol 1973;89:3–9.
13. Johnson LN, Wall M. Automated perimetry in neuro-ophthalmology. In Focal Points, Clinical Modules for Ophthalmologists. Am Acad Ophthalmol 1993;8:1–11.
14. Carroll FD. Nutritional amblyopia. Arch Ophthalmol 1966;76:406–411.
15. Carroll FD. The etiology and treatment of tobacco-alcohol amblyopia. Part I. Am J Ophthalmol 1944;27:713–725.
16. Golnik KC, Schaible ER. Folate-responsive optic neuropathy. J Neuro-ophthalmol 1994;14:163–169.
17. Foulds WS, Chilholm IA, Bronte-Stewart J, Wilson TM. Vitamin B-12 absorption in tobacco amblyopia. Br J Ophthalmol 1969;53:393–397.
18. Foulds WS, Chilholm IA, Bronte-Stewart J, Wilson TM. The optic neuropathy of pernicious anemia. Arch Ophthalmol 1969;82:427–432.
19. Miller NR. Walsh and Hoyt's Clinical Neuro-Ophthalmology (4th ed). Vol. 1. Baltimore, MD: Williams & Wilkins, 192;254–260, 289–307.
20. Keltner JL, Johnson CA, Spurr JO, et al. Baseline profile of optic neuritis. Arch Ophthalmol 1993;111:231–234.
21. Keltner JL, Johnson CA, Spurr JO, et al. Visual field profile of optic neuritis one year follow-up in the Optic Neuritis Treatment Trial. Arch Ophthalmol 1994;112:946–953.
22. Hayreh SS. Anterior ischaemic optic neuropathy. I. Terminology and pathogenesis. Br J Ophthalmol 1974;58:955–963.
23. Boghen DR, Glaser JS. Ischaemic optic neuropathy. The clinical profile and natural history. Brain 1975;98:689–708.
24. Cullen JF. Ischemic optic neuropathy. Trans Ophthalmol Soc UK 1967;87: 759–774.
25. Borchert M, Lessell S. Progressive and recurrent non-arteritic anterior ischemic optic neuropathy. Am J Ophthalmol 1988;106:443–449.
26. Corbett JJ, Savino PJ, Thompson HS, et al. Visual loss in pseudotumor cerebri. Follow-up of 57 patients from five to 41 years and a profile of 14 patients with severe visual loss. Arch Neurol 1982;39:461–474.
27. Smith TJ, Baker RS. Perimetric findings in pseudotumor cerebri using automated techniques. Ophthalmology 1986;93:887–894.
28. Boddie HG, Banna M, Bradley WG. "Benign" intracranial hypertension. Brain 1974;97:313–326.
29. Savino PJ, Glaser JS, Rosenberg MA. A clinical analysis of pseudopapilledema. II. Visual field defects. Arch Ophthalmol 1979;97:71–75.
30. Mosier MA, Lieberman MF, Green WR, Knox DL. Hypoplasia of the optic nerve. Arch Ophthalmol 1978;96:1437–1442.
31. Frisen L. Visual Field Defects due to Hypoplasia of the Optic Nerve. In EL Greve (ed), Third International Visual Field Symposium. (Doc Ophthalmol Proc Ser;19.) The Hague, Dr. W Junk, 1979;81–86.
32. Hollenhorst RW, Young BR. Ocular Manifestations Produced by Adenomas of the Pituitary Gland: Analysis of 1,000 Cases. In PO Kohler, GT Ross (eds), Diagnosis and Treatment of Pituitary Tumors. Amsterdam: Excerpta Medica, 1973;53–68.

33. Cannavo S, De Natale R, Princi P, et al. Effectiveness of computer-assisted perimetry in the diagnosis of pituitary adenomas. Clin Endocrinol 1989;31: 673–678.
34. De Natale R, Cannavo S. Computerized perimetry in the early diagnosis of hypophyseal microadenoma. Acta XXV Concilium Ophthalmologicum. Proceedings of the XXVth International Congress of Ophthalmology. Rome, May 4-10, 1986. Amsterdam: Kugler, 1987:1748–1751.
35. Grochowicki M, Vighetto A, Berquet S, et al. Pituitary adenomas: automatic static perimetry and Goldmann perimetry. A comparative study of 345 visual field charts. Br J Ophthalmol 1991;75:219–221.
36. Smith JL. Homonymous hemianopia: a review of one hundred cases. Am J Ophthalmol 1962;54:616–622.
37. Bell RA, Thompson HS. Relative afferent pupillary defect in optic tract hemianopias. Am J Ophthalmol 1978;85:538–540.
38. Bender MB, Bodis-Wollner I. Visual dysfunctions in optic tract lesions. Ann Neurol 1978;3:187–193.
39. Frisén L, Holmegaard L, Rosencrantz M. Sectorial optic atrophy and homonymous, horizontal sectoranopia: a lateral choroidal artery syndrome? J Neurol Neurosurg Psychiatry 1978;41:374–380.
40. Frisen L. Quadruple sectoranopia and sectorial optic atrophy: a syndrome of the distal anterior choroidal artery. J Neurol Neurosurg Psychiatry 1979;42: 590–594.
41. Miller NM. Walsh and Joyt's Clinical Neuro-Ophthalmology (4th ed). Baltimore: Williams & Wilkins, 1982;134.
42. Cogan DG. Neurology of the Visual System. Springfield, IL: Charles C. Thomas, 1966;254.
43. Gray LG, Galetta SL, Siegal T, Schatz NJ. The central visual field in homonymous hemianopia. Arch Neurol 1997;54:312–317.
44. Smith CG, Richardson WFG. The course and distribution of the arteries supplying the visual (striate) cortex. Am J Ophthalmol 1966;61:1391–1396.
45. Stewart JFG. Automated perimetry and malingerers. Can the Humphrey be outwitted? Ophthalmology 1995;102:27–31.

4

Systemic Neurologic Evaluation

When examining patients with ocular manifestations of neurologic disease, it is often necessary to do additional neurologic testing to obtain further insight into a patient's condition. Such testing is simple but requires a general understanding of some basic neurologic concepts. A neurologic screening done as an adjunct to an ocular examination should not take the place of a comprehensive examination that would be done by a neurologist. Nonetheless, it provides useful clinical information regarding the nature of a neuro-ophthalmic disturbance.

The indications for a neurologic assessment in the eye care setting are numerous. Any neurologic disorder that affects the brain has the potential to produce visual signs and symptoms that are manifested by cranial nerve palsies, nystagmus and other motility disturbances, visual field defects, transient visual loss, papilledema, and pupillary disturbances. The optometrist faced with such a presentation is obligated to manage the patient by evaluating the problem and ordering an appropriate workup or by making an appropriate referral. In many instances, a neurologic assessment will reveal whether a presenting sign or symptom has other neurologic associations that will help localize the source of the problem to a specific region of the brain. Such localization is important in ordering accurate neuroimaging studies.

As has been emphasized throughout these chapters, the history plays an important role in evaluating patients with neurologic signs and symptoms. An acute onset of symptoms suggests a vascular or ischemic etiology; a progressive onset of symptoms suggests a structural defect such as a tumor or degenerative disease. In many instances, patients presenting with a neuro-ophthalmic sign or symptom will be able to report an associated neurologic deficit, and the examiner simply uses the neurologic screening to confirm it. This is particularly true in an outpatient, optometric setting, where patients are ambulatory and healthier than those in inpatient, hospital settings.

A neurologic screening takes only a few minutes and consists of the following parts[1-3]: mental status assessment, cranial nerve assessment, motor assessment, assessment of reflexes, coordination, and sensory assessment.

Mental Status Assessment

Much of this assessment begins in the history taking part of the examination. As mentioned previously, history taking in neuro-ophthalmic disease is thorough and detailed. During the extensive period of questioning, the examiner should take note of the patient's level of alertness, which is gauged by the patient's ability to comprehend questions and to provide accurate and meaningful information. Whenever possible, information from family members and close friends should be obtained. Many patients will deny a history of memory loss or neurologic difficulty, but information from family members may suggest otherwise. Depending on the information provided by the patient during the history, a decision to do a formal assessment of mental status can be made. Of particular importance in a mental status assessment is memory, particularly recent memory, which tends to be affected earlier in neurologic disease processes.

■ Performing the Test

Orientation to Time and Place

Even a relatively alert patient can be somewhat disoriented to time and place. Orientation to time includes asking the patient to report the current year, month, and day, whereas orientation to place involves asking the patient where he or she is (doctor's office), followed by what town, state, country, and so on.

General Information

The patient should be able to state his or her full name, as well as that of anyone who may be accompanying the patient. In addition, some basic current events such as "Who is the president of the United States?" should be asked.

Memory and Concentration

The patient is asked to spell a five-letter word. If the patient can do this, he or she is next asked to spell it backward. An inability to spell a word backward suggests an organic mental deficit. The degree of the deficit can be quantified by having the patient spell three- and four-letter words forward and backward. Difficulty suggests impaired immediate recall. If the patient is illiterate, he or she can be asked to repeat a numbered sequence or to count backward from 100 by 3s. To test intermediate recall, the patient is given three objects to remember (e.g., coffee, taxi, telephone) and is asked to repeat them several minutes later.

Interpretation

The cognitive function tested in the mental status examination is governed mainly by the frontal lobes. Abnormalities in mental status suggest dementia, which can have many possible etiologies. Among these are cerebrovascular disease, alcoholism, head trauma, central nervous system infection, nutritional deficiencies, and neurodegenerative diseases.

Cranial Nerve Testing

Of the 12 cranial nerves, six are directly involved in sensory, motor, or autonomic input to the eye.[4] Cranial nerve dysfunction can occur in conjunction with cortical or brain stem disease, or it may occur in isolation.

■ Performing the Test for Cranial Nerve I

The function of cranial nerve I (the olfactory nerve) is sensation of olfaction or smell.

Testing should be done with a mild, nonirritating aroma. Tobacco and mild soaps or spices are ideal. Irritating agents such as alcohol or ammonia should not be used because they stimulate the intranasal pain endings of the trigeminal nerve rather than the olfactory nerve. Each nostril should be tested separately with at least two different agents. The patient closes his or her eyes and is asked to identify the fragrance (Figure 4.1).

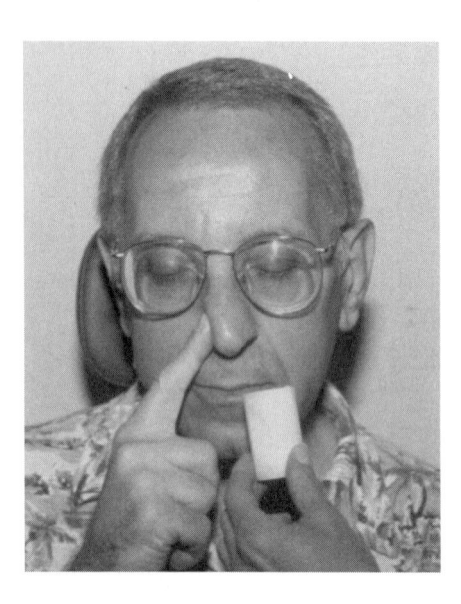

Figure 4.1
Testing olfaction. The patient closes his or her eyes and occludes one nostril so that each side is tested separately.

Interpretation

Anosmia (loss of smell) can occur with upper respiratory infections, diabetes, or compressive disease involving the olfactory bulbs.[5] It may also be seen after head trauma.[6]

■ Performing the Test for Cranial Nerve II

The function of cranial nerve II (the optic nerve) is the conveyance of special sensory visual information from the retina.

Optic nerve assessment is well known to the optometrist and is part of the routine eye examination. Tests of optic nerve function include visual acuity, color vision, pupil testing, and visual field testing. Ophthalmoscopy should also be included to visualize the optic nerve head in the posterior pole. Optic nerve disease may be unilateral or bilateral; therefore, each eye should be tested separately.

Interpretation

Reductions in visual acuity are commonly seen with optic nerve disease, but they are also seen in patients with refractive errors, medial opacities, corneal disease, and retinal disease. Reductions in color vision are seen in unilateral or bilateral optic nerve disease, as are visual field defects. Ophthalmoscopically, pallor, abnormal vasculature, or swelling are common manifestations of optic nerve disease. Swelling, when bilateral and associated with normal optic nerve function, is indicative of increased intracranial pressure rather than primary optic nerve disease.

■ Performing the Test for Cranial Nerves III, IV, and VI

The function of cranial nerve III (the oculomotor nerve) is the control of extraocular muscles, including the levator, superior rectus, inferior rectus, inferior oblique, and medial rectus. Cranial nerve III also innervates the iris sphincter and ciliary body, resulting in pupillary constriction and accommodation. Cranial nerve IV (the trochlear nerve) controls the superior oblique muscle. Cranial nerve VI (the abducens nerve) controls the lateral rectus muscle.

Evaluation of cranial nerves III, IV, and VI involves ocular motility testing and is discussed in detail in Chapter 1. In a neurologic screening examination, the patient is instructed to follow a target that is moved through the seven diagnostic positions of gaze. Limitation of a particular extraocular muscle is noted by observing a restriction or when the patient reports diplopia. An assessment of pupillary constriction to light and near and eyelid position is also necessary to fully evaluate cranial nerve III.

■ Performing the Test for Cranial Nerve V

The function of cranial nerve V (the trigeminal nerve) includes a motor component to the muscles of mastication and a sensory component to the face, eye, and other intracranial structures.

To test the motor component, the examiner palpates the jaw muscles while the patient's teeth are clenched. Next, the examiner watches while the patient slowly opens his or her mouth, observing any deviation to one side.

To test the sensory component, the examiner lightly touches both sides of the forehead, cheeks, and chin simultaneously with a pin, tissue, or fingers, and the patient reports any perceived difference between the two sides. The corneal reflex can be tested by lightly touching the cornea of first the right and then the left eye with a cotton swab twisted to a point.

Interpretation

A difference of muscle strength on one side on teeth clenching or a deviation of the jaw on mouth opening indicates a motor deficit. The sensory component of the trigeminal nerve has three branches that supply different parts of the face: The ophthalmic division (V1) supplies the forehead and eye, the maxillary division (V2) supplies the cheeks, and the mandibular division (V3) supplies the chin. A perceived difference in light touch on one side relative to the other indicates a sensory deficit in that dermatome. The corneal reflex requires both an intact sensory component of the trigeminal nerve but also an intact facial nerve. When the cornea of one eye is touched, both eyes should blink.

■ Performing the Test for Cranial Nerve VII

Cranial nerve VII (the facial nerve) has a motor component to the muscles of facial expression and to the stapedius muscle of the middle ear. Visceral motor (lacrimal and other glands), as well as general sensory and special sensory components, are also part of this nerve.

Screening of facial nerve function emphasizes the motor component. The examiner begins by observing the patient's facial tone, paying careful attention to the degree and symmetry of brow wrinkling, symmetry of the palpebral apertures, and presence of the nasolabial fold and position of the mouth. The patient is then asked to smile, close the eyes, raise the eyebrows, and blow out the cheeks or whistle.

Interpretation

A weakness of the upper and lower halves of the face is typical of a lower motor neuron, or peripheral, facial nerve palsy (Bell's palsy). Upper motor neuron involvement affects the cerebral cortex or its input to the facial nucleus in the pons and results in weakness of one side of the mouth with no significant involvement of the brow or eyelids. This occurs because cortical or upper motor neuron innervation to the upper half of the face is bilateral, whereas innervation to the bottom of the face is unilateral.

■ Performing the Test for Cranial Nerve VIII

Cranial nerve VIII (the acoustic nerve) transmits information regarding hearing (cochlear division) and balance (vestibular division) to the brain stem from the inner ear.

Gross testing of hearing is accomplished by placing a stimulus adjacent to the ear on either side and asking the patient if there is any perceived difference in loudness. Appropriate stimuli include a ticking watch or two fingers rubbed together.

Interpretation

A reduction in hearing may occur from a conduction deficit or sensorineural deficit. To differentiate between the two, the examiner simply asks the patient to hum. If the humming is heard louder on the side with the reduced hearing, the deficit is with conduction. If the humming is louder on the side with normal hearing, the hearing loss is sensorineural. Conduction deficits are commonly seen in patients with earwax or middle ear disease, whereas sensorineural deafness occurs with lesions in the cochlea, the nerve itself, or in the eighth nerve nucleus in the brain stem. Disease of the vestibular component results in nystagmus and vertigo, the latter often manifesting itself by disturbances of gait and coordination.

■ Performing the Test for Cranial Nerve IX and X

Cranial nerves IX and X have both motor and sensory components. The motor components of cranial nerves IX (the glossopharyngeal nerve) and X (the vagus nerve) are emphasized during screening evaluations. Cranial nerve IX innervates the stylopharyngeus muscle; cranial nerve X controls muscles of the palate, pharynx, and larynx.

The examiner should listen to the patient's voice, noting any nasal quality or hoarseness. Next, movement of the uvula is observed as the patient opens his or her mouth and says "ahh." A tongue depressor facilitates observation of the uvula. The gag reflex is then tested while the tongue is depressed by touching the soft palate or pharynx with a cotton swab, with the examiner observing whether the soft palate retracts symmetrically.

Interpretation

Pharyngeal weakness results in a nasal quality to the patient's voice, whereas laryngeal weakness results in hoarseness. If the uvula does not move up centrally when the patient says "ahh," bilateral palatal muscle paresis is suggested. If it deviates to one side, a contralateral vagus lesion is suggested. If the uvula moves on saying "ahh" but not with the gag reflex, a glossopharyngeal deficit is indicated; however, this is extremely rare and the gag reflex can generally be omitted.[7]

■ Performing the Test for Cranial Nerve XI

Cranial nerve XI (the accessory nerve) is a motor nerve that innervates the sternocleidomastoid and trapezius muscles.

The patient is instructed to turn his or her face against the manual resistance of the examiner's hand on either side. The patient is then asked to shrug his or her shoulders against the manual resistance of the examiner (Figure 4.2).

Interpretation

Weakness on the face turn indicates weakness of the sternocleidomastoid muscle, whereas a difference on shoulder shrugging indicates weakness of the trapezius muscles.

■ Performing the Test for Cranial Nerve XII

Cranial nerve XII (the hypoglossal nerve) is a motor nerve that supplies all of the muscles of the tongue except the palatoglossus muscle. The patient is instructed to stick out his or her tongue while the examiner observes any deviation. Next, the patient is instructed to push his or her tongue into the cheek. The examiner notes the strength of the tongue while pushing against the cheek (Figure 4.3).

Figure 4.2
Accessory nerve testing. To test sternocleidomastoid function, the patient turns his or her head against the examiner's resistance (A). To test trapezius function, the patient shrugs his or her shoulders against the manual resistance of the examiner (B).

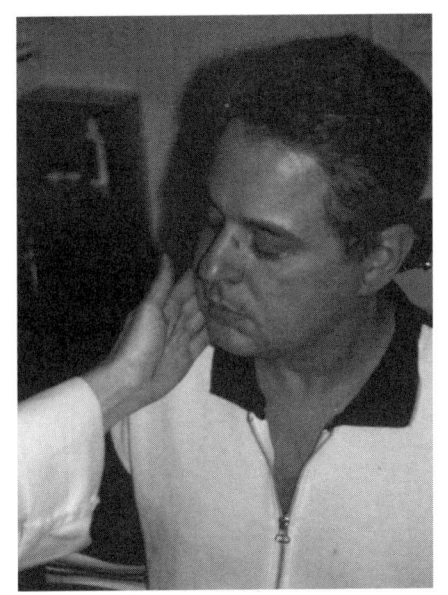

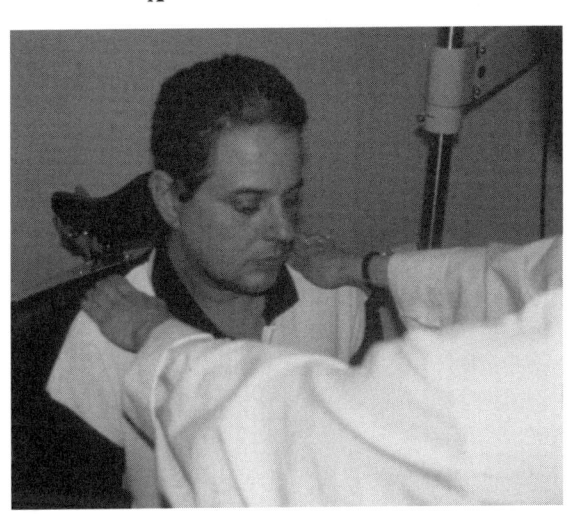

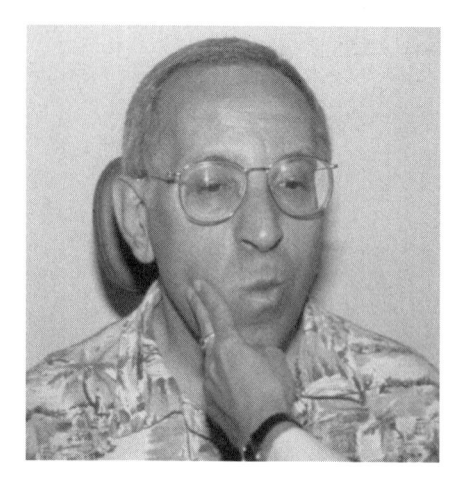

Figure 4.3
One test of hypoglossal nerve function is to instruct the patient to push the tongue into his or her cheek. The examiner notes its strength by pushing against it through the cheek.

Interpretation

A deviation of the tongue to either side or a relative weakness on one side suggests a lesion along the ipsilateral nerve pathway.

Motor Examination

The corticospinal pathway is the motor pathway to the upper and lower extremities. The upper motor neurons of the corticospinal tract synapse in the spinal cord; therefore, intracranial disease that affects the corticospinal pathway results in upper motor neuron involvement. This is an important concept because upper and lower motor neuron diseases have different clinical presentations. Signs of upper motor neuron disease result in increased muscle tone or spastic muscle paralysis and in exaggerated tendon reflexes. Lower motor neuron disease results in paralysis with loss of muscle tone or flaccid paralysis, loss of tendon reflexes, and fasciculations.

Central nervous system disease that results in ocular involvement can occur with cortical, brain stem, and cerebellar disease. Therefore, motor pathways that may be involved include the upper and lower motor neurons of the cranial nerves and the upper motor neurons of the corticospinal tract. Motor function seen in such disease therefore consists of cranial nerve deficits and motor weakness of the upper and lower extremities. The motor examination in screening of patients with neuro-ophthalmic disease is based on testing for relative right-left weakness of the upper and lower extremities in addition to cranial nerve testing.

■ Upper and Lower Extremity Drift

The patient closes his or her eyes and holds the hands out in front, parallel to the floor and with palms facing upward. The examiner observes for 15–30 seconds, looking for changes in arm position. The lower extremity can be tested by having the patient lie on his or her stomach, with the knees flexed at a 90-degree angle. The examiner observes any changes in leg position.

Interpretation

When testing upper and lower extremity drift, there should be no significant change in arm or leg position after 15–30 seconds. If one arm pronates and drifts downward, weakness is suspected on that side. Bilateral weakness is suggested if both arms drift downward. Ipsilateral cerebellar disease is suggested if one arm rises. Weakness of the lower extremity is evident if the leg on the weak side wavers, drops, or both. An upper motor neuron deficit will result in weakness contralateral to the side of the lesion.

■ Other Tests of Upper and Lower Extremity Strength

To evaluate the upper extremity, the examiner grips the patient's right hand with his or her right hand. The patient is asked to pull the examiner's hand toward himself or herself against the examiner's resistance (Figure 4.4A). The same is repeated with the left side. The patient is then instructed to grasp the examiner's right middle and index fingers with the right hand tightly while the examiner attempts to pull his or her fingers out. The same is repeated on the left side. To test the lower extremity, the patient is asked raise one knee against the manual resistance of the examiner (Figure 4.4B). Next, the patient is instructed to flex the foot against the manual resistance of the examiner. Disruption of the upper motor neurons of the corticospinal tract would result in a contralateral weakness.

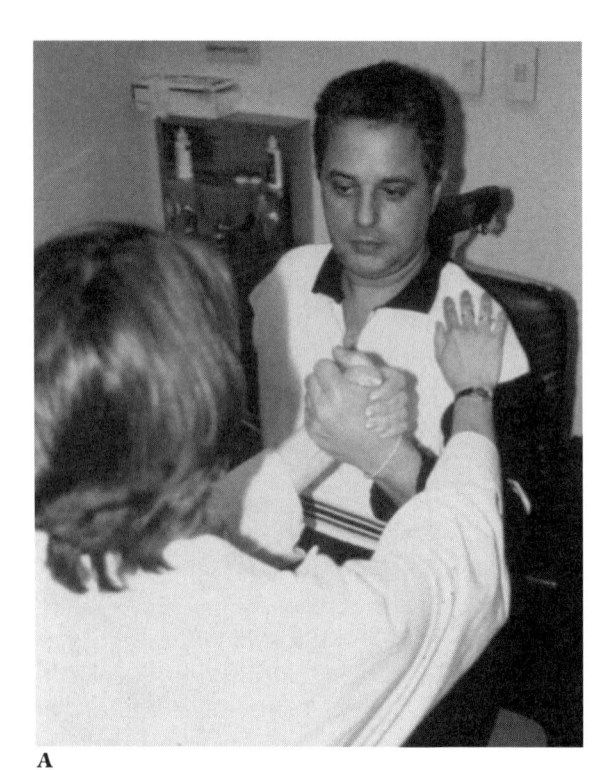

Figure 4.4
(A) To test motor function of the upper extremity, the patient pulls the examiner's hand toward himself or herself against the examiner's manual resistance. (B) The lower extremity is evaluated by asking the patient to raise his or her leg against the examiner's resistance.

Sensory Evaluation

Intracranial lesions of the cerebrum or brain stem will typically result in generalized sensory losses of the contralateral upper and lower extremities; therefore, in patients with neuro-ophthalmic disease, it is necessary to do only a gross sensory examination of the face, hands, and feet. Sensory evaluation consists of testing of the primary sensory modalities, which include pain, proprioception, stereognosis, vibration, and light touch.

■ Evaluating Pain

The patient is seated with eyes closed, hands in lap palms down. The examiner places a sharp stimulus on the dorsum of each hand and asks the patient if it feels sharp or dull. The same is repeated with the dorsum

B

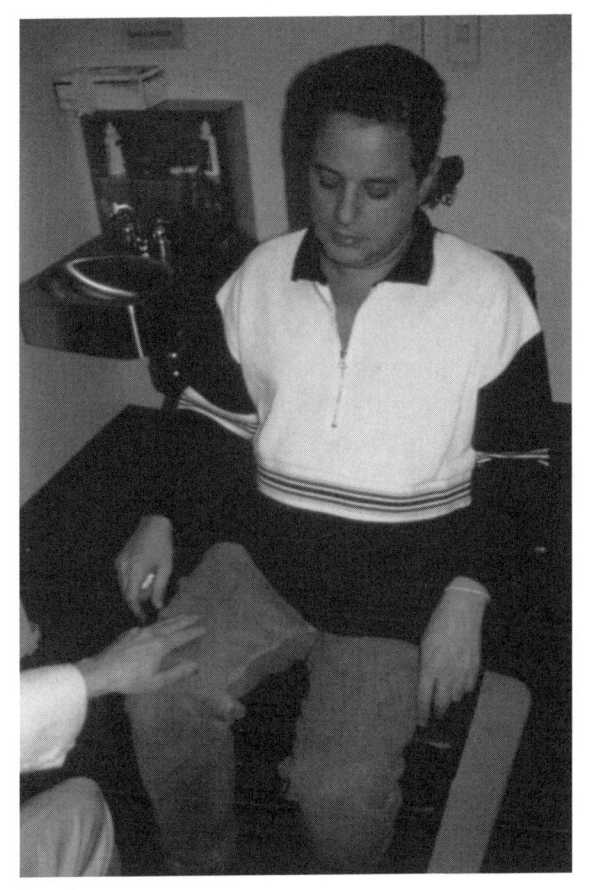

of each foot and on either side of the face. A broken stick of a cotton-tipped applicator is ideal because it can be discarded after each patient. The pointed part of the broken stick provides a sharp stimulus, whereas the cotton-tipped end provides a dull stimulus.

■ Evaluating Temperature

Ask the patient if an ophthalmoscope handle feels cool or warm when touched to the hands, feet, and cheeks. Likewise, a wooden tongue depressor will be perceived as a warm stimulus.

Evaluating Proprioception and Position

With the patient's eyes closed, the big toe is grasped from the sides to avoid clues elicited by pressure. The toe is bent upward or downward, and the patient is asked to report whether the toe is "up" or "down." Testing of the upper extremity is unnecessary if the lower extremity is normal.

Light Touch

If pain and proprioception are intact, it is not necessary to test light touch as it is unlikely to be affected. Double, simultaneous stimulation of the dorsum of the hands, feet, and cheeks is done with a cotton wisp and the patient compares the sensation on either side.

Interpretation

Brain stem lesions produce hemisensory deficits on the ipsilateral side of the face and contralateral upper and lower extremities. Parietal lobe disease and thalamic lesions result in hemisensory deficits of the contralateral face and contralateral upper and lower extremities.

Coordination and Balance

The cerebellum and basal ganglia play an important role in coordination. In addition, balance is important to coordination, and because vision, proprioception, and vestibular sense all feed directly or indirectly into the cerebellum, they play an important role in balance and coordination.

Testing Coordination

Finger-to-Nose Test

The patient closes his or her eyes and extends the arms out at his or her sides and parallel to the floor. The patient is instructed to alternately touch his or her right and left index fingers to the nose quickly and repetitively in succession.

Heel-to-Shin Test

The seated patient is instructed to place his or her right heel on his or her left shin at the knee and move it down the length of the shin to the ankle and back up to the knee again. The same is repeated on the opposite side.

Rapid Alternating Hand and Foot Movements

The patient is instructed to alternately touch his or her thumb with each fingertip or to rapidly flip-flop one hand while it rests on the other. Rapid foot movements are elicited by instructing the patient to rapidly tap his or her foot to the floor while the heel rests in place.

Interpretation

On finger-to-nose and heel-to-shin testing, cerebellar dysfunction is indicated when the finger over- or undershoots its target (dysmetria) or when a tremor develops as the finger approaches its target. If a tremor improves with movement and is more apparent at rest (resting tremor), basal ganglia disease is suggested (Parkinson's disease). On heel-to-shin testing, cerebellar dysfunction is indicated when the heel falls off the shin or if the knee wobbles from side to side. Difficulty on rapid alternating hand and foot movements is indicative of ipsilateral cerebellar disease.

■ Testing Balance

Tandem gait and the Romberg test are key tests for balance. To test tandem gait, the patient is instructed to walk, placing one foot directly in front of the other, heel to toe (Figure 4.5). Normal patients are able to walk without swaying. The Romberg test is simply tandem walking that is done with the eyes closed, and this is done when tandem walking is normal to assist in differentiating the cause of the balance problem.

Interpretation

If the patient has difficulty performing tandem walking with the eyes open, cerebellar disease is indicated. If proprioception is lacking, the

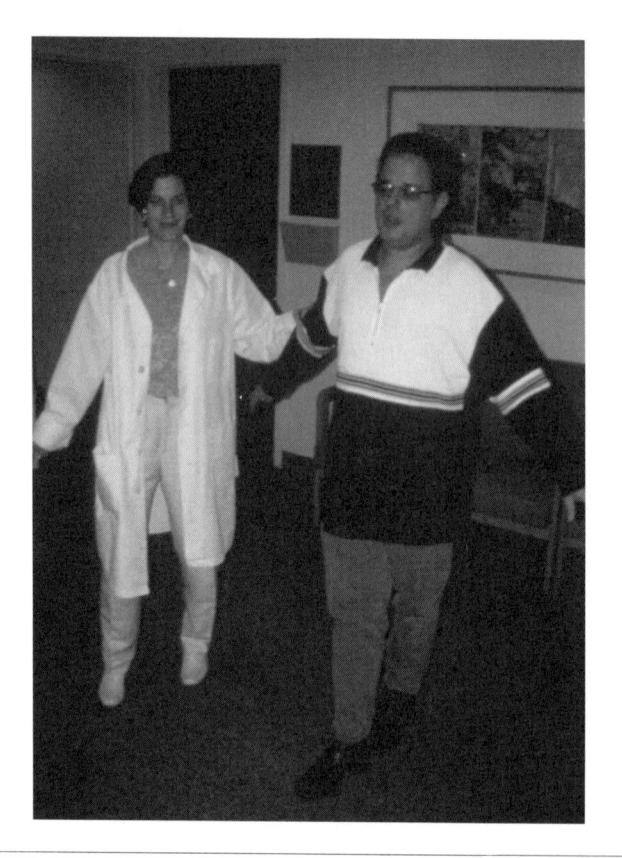

Figure 4.5 A key test for balance is tandem gait. The patient demonstrates this by walking heel-to-toe while the examiner stands close by to assist the patient if necessary.

patient will keep his or her balance with the eyes open but not with the eyes closed. This occurs because vision, vestibular sense, and proprioception—all of which have cerebellar connections—are involved in balance and two of the three must be functioning normally to maintain balance. The Romberg test eliminates visual input; therefore, if a patient cannot tandem walk with the eyes closed, the proprioception or vestibular sense must be faulty. Vestibular disease is suspected when the patient complains of vertigo and is typically manifested by nystagmus. If the patient has no vertigo or nystagmus, proprioception must be faulty.

Reflexes

The major reflexes can be easily elicited and include triceps, biceps, knee jerk, ankle jerk, and the Babinski sign.

The reflex hammer is held loosely with the fingers rather than with the whole hand. The patient is instructed to relax. The appropriate tendon is struck lightly but firmly with the reflex hammer.

Triceps

The arm is placed across the chest with the elbow at a 90-degree angle. The triceps tendon is struck just above the elbow and the triceps muscle is observed for the contraction.

Biceps

The patient's hands are placed on his abdomen. The examiner's index finger is placed on the biceps tendon at the bend of the elbow. The hammer is swung directly onto the finger while observing the biceps muscle for contraction (Figure 4.6).

Knee Jerk

The patient is seated with the knees at a 90-degree angle. The patellar tendon is struck directly, just below the patella. The quadriceps muscle in the thigh is observed or felt through a heavily clothed patient for contraction.

Ankle Jerk

The foot is held at 90 degrees. The Achilles' tendon is struck directly and the calf muscles are observed for contraction.

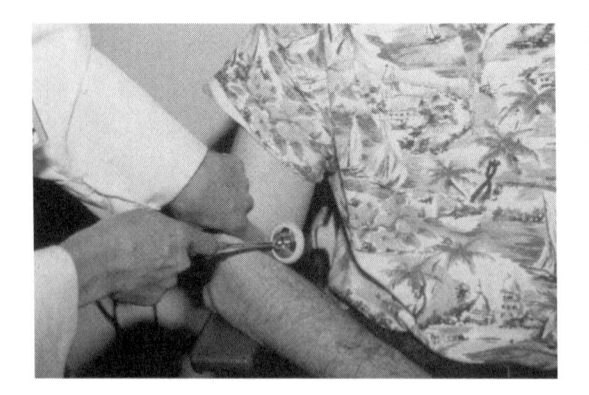

Figure 4.6
To elicit the biceps reflex, the examiner places his or her index finger firmly over the biceps tendon at the bend of the elbow. The hammer makes contact directly onto the examiner's finger.

■ Interpretation of the Triceps, Biceps, Knee Jerk, and Ankle Jerk Reflexes

A normal person may exhibit a wide range of reflexes from active to absent; therefore, asymmetric responses are more important indicators of pathology. Increased reflexes are seen in upper motor neuron lesions, and reduced or absent reflexes are seen in lower motor neuron disease or peripheral neuropathies. Disorders of neuro-ophthalmic significance are more likely to result in upper motor neuron deficits with increased reflexes on the impaired side. Disorders that commonly result in decreased tendon reflexes include Adie's tonic pupil.

■ Babinski Reflex (Plantar Response)

Shoes and socks are removed. The foot is elevated and supported with the examiner's hand or knee. The examiner gently but firmly draws a pointed object, such as the end of a wooden cotton-tipped applicator, up the lateral portion of the bottom of the foot from the heel forward and across the footpad.

Interpretation of the Babinski Reflex

A normal response is plantar flexion of the toes. A positive result is dorsiflexion of the big toe with a fanning out or spreading of the other toes, which indicates upper motor neuron disease.

Cerebrovascular Disease and Stroke

In many instances, neuro-ophthalmic presentations are the result of cerebrovascular disease and stroke. When a completed stroke occurs, the neuro-ophthalmic sequelae are numerous and include both afferent and efferent disturbances. The optometrist plays an important role in the care of stroke patients by recognizing the visual system deficits and in addressing them through the rehabilitative process. In other instances, an ocular finding may be the first manifestation of cerebrovascular disease. It is important for the optometrist to recognize potential signs of cerebrovascular disease and alert the primary physician. This ensures prompt medical intervention so that the future risk of stroke is minimized.

Blood is supplied to the brain by an anterior and posterior circulation. The anterior circulation is composed of the internal carotid arteries and their branches and supplies most of the cerebral cortex, basal ganglia, internal capsule, and optic radiations. The posterior circulation consists of the vertebrobasilar system and its branches and supplies the brain stem, cerebellum, thalamus, and parts of the temporal and occipital lobes. The ocular manifestations of cerebrovascular disease are numerous and characterized by the circulation involved (Table 4.1).[8]

Cerebrovascular disease results in damage to brain tissue from ischemia or, less commonly, hemorrhage. Ischemia occurs by a number of mechanisms. Thrombosis of large cerebral vessels usually occurs from atherosclerosis and can result in occlusion of the internal carotid and vertebral and basilar arteries and their branches. Less commonly, infection or inflammatory disease can result in thrombosis. The resulting cerebrovas-

Table 4.1 Ocular Manifestations of Cerebrovascular Disease

Anterior Circulation	Posterior Circulation
Amaurosis fugax	Homonymous hemianopia
Retinal vascular occlusive disease (Color Plate 15)	Extraocular muscle palsies
Homonymous hemianopia	Gaze palsies and related disorders
Ocular ischemic syndrome	Nystagmus and ocular dysmetria
Cranial nerve palsies	Bilateral transient vision loss

cular manifestation depends on the vessel involved and the integrity of its collateral circulation. Lacunar infarctions are small infarctions that occur from occlusion of small, deep penetrating arteries. They occur most commonly in the deep portions of the brain, and in the pons and posterior limb of the internal capsule but can also occur in the cerebral white matter, cerebellum, and anterior limb of the internal capsule. Embolic disease occurs when an atherosclerotic plaque breaks off and travels distally to occlude a smaller artery. Emboli can also originate in the heart, and the cardiac abnormalities that produce them are numerous.[9]

Hemorrhagic mechanisms of cerebrovascular disease are much less common than ischemic mechanisms. Hypertension is the most common cause of cerebral hemorrhage, but other etiologies include vascular malformations, infectious diseases, and drug and alcohol abuse. Although intracranial hemorrhage occurs much less commonly, it makes up a much greater percentage of cerebrovascular accidents in younger patients, who are far less prone to ischemic mechanisms.

Many patients, particularly those with atherosclerotic disease, will manifest early warning signs of stroke. Warning signs include transient ischemic attacks (TIAs), which are episodes of focal cerebral dysfunction that completely resolve within 24 hours and usually less than 30 minutes. Amaurosis fugax is a form of TIA confined to the retina, which results in transient blindness of one eye that typically lasts 5 minutes. Observation of the patient's fundus may reveal an embolus that originated from more proximal vasculature in the carotid arteries or the heart (Color Plate 15).

When a completed stroke occurs, the resulting damage to brain tissue is permanent. Therefore, the most important way to combat stroke is by recognizing the early, transient warning signs and ocular manifestations of cerebrovascular disease and, perhaps even more important, identifying that the patient is at risk for stroke. As many as 80% of all strokes are preventable because they result from modifiable risk factors.[10] Risk factors for cerebrovascular disease and stroke are summarized in Table 4.2.

Because the prevention of stroke is an important aspect of cerebrovascular disease management, the optometrist plays an important role as a primary provider in the health care system. Optometric responsibilities of stroke prevention are geared toward recognition of cerebrovascular risk factors and the ocular manifestations of cerebrovascular disease. The best way to accomplish this is through a comprehensive examination that includes blood pressure testing. A careful history will also reveal important risk factors. Recognition of signs requires thorough knowledge

Table 4.2 Risk Factors for Cerebrovascular Disease and Stroke

Age
Sex
Hypertension*
Heart disease*
Smoking*
Hyperlipidemia*
Heavy alcohol use*

*Indicates modifiable risk factor.

of the ocular manifestations of cerebrovascular disease and an understanding of potential sources and an appropriate workup.

Billing and Reimbursement

There is no appropriate Current Procedural Terminology that applies to neurologic screening techniques. Although these tests do not have standalone procedure codes, they may justify billing a higher level of office code due to the extra time spent on the examination.

Related International Classification of Diseases-9 (ICD-9) Terminology

Olfactory nerve disorder	352.0
Trigeminal nerve disorder	350.9
Facial palsy	351.0
Multiple cranial nerve palsy	352.6

References

1. Weiner WJ, Goetz CG (eds). Neurology for the Non-Neurologist (3rd ed). Philadelphia: Lippincott–Raven, 1994.

2. Simon RP, Aminoff MJ, Greenberg DA. Clinical Neurology. Norwalk, CT: Appleton & Lange, 1989.
3. Bernat JL, Vincent FM. Neurology: Problems in Primary Care. Oradell, NJ: Medical Economics, 1987.
4. Wilson-Pauwels L, Akesson EJ, Stewart PA. Cranial Nerves: Anatomy and Clinical Comments. Philadelphia: BC Decker, 1988.
5. Rowland LP (ed). Merrit's Textbook of Neurology (9th ed). Baltimore: Williams & Wilkins, 1995.
6. Friedman AP, Merritt HH. Damage to cranial nerves resulting from head injury. Bull Los Angeles Neurol Soc 1944;9:135–139.
7. Goldberg S. The Four-Minute Neurologic Exam. Miami: MedMaster, 1989.
8. Hollenhorst RW. Carotid and vertebral-basilar arterial stenosis and occlusion: neuro-ophthalmologic considerations. Trans Am Acad Ophthalmol Otolaryngol 1962;66:166–180.
9. Helgason CM, Sherman DG. Neurologic manifestations of cardiac disease. Neurol Clin 1989;7:469–488.
10. Gorelick PB. Stroke prevention: an opportunity for efficient utilization of health care resources during the coming decade. Stroke 1994;25:220–224.

5

Additional Neuro-Ophthalmic Testing

In a routine eye examination, tests of visual function are conducted to determine whether the visual system functions normally. In patients with neuro-ophthalmic disease, a determination of some abnormality has already been made. Tests of visual function are then used to identify which part of the system is functioning abnormally. It is also important to know the degree of abnormal function for monitoring purposes.

■
Color Vision Testing

Loss of color vision is a common occurrence in patients with visual pathway disease and is therefore an important aspect of neuro-ophthalmic diagnosis. It is generally accepted that diseases of the retina are characterized by loss of blue-yellow discrimination, and optic nerve disease results in red-green defects.[1] Exceptions to this rule are well known. In the case of optic nerve disease, color vision defects really depend on the type of visual field defect associated with them. Red-green defects in optic nerve disease are most pronounced when the papillomacular bundles are involved[1] and there is characteristic acuity loss. If acuity is spared, blue-yellow defects are more likely.[2] Therefore, clinical tests of color vision (Color Plate 16) used in neuro-ophthalmic disease should be capable of detecting both types of defects.

A number of color vision tests are available for in-office use. Pseudoisochromatic plates[3] (PIPs) are the most popular; the Ishihara series is the most widely used. In testing color vision with these plates, the examiner must realize that most of the PIPs are geared mainly toward diagnosing congenital defects of the red-green type. However, because most acquired color defects seen in neuro-ophthalmic disease are also of the red-green type, they are still useful if used with caution, as many patients with acquired color defects will pass color testing with PIPs. Although different types of commercially available PIPs vary in different ways, all of them rely on the patient's ability to detect a figure against a background of confusing hues. Each system comes with its own set of directions and scoring system, but a number of rules apply universally:

1. Testing for acquired color vision defects must be done monocularly.
2. Appropriate illumination is required.
3. The patient is allowed just a few seconds per page, although spontaneous corrections are allowed.
4. The patient is tested at reading distance with the appropriate reading correction.

■ Interpretation

The scoring system available with PIPs should be used with caution when evaluating patients with acquired color vision defects. Many patients with acquired color vision defects are able to make correct responses, albeit with difficulty, and are inappropriately graded as normal. The examiner should note whether the patient has difficulty with one or both eyes. Patients who are noted to have difficulty despite having correct responses should be investigated with more sensitive tests of color vision.

Color Sorting Tests

Another popular type of color vision test is one that involves color sorting. Tests of color sorting require the patient to arrange a group of colored caps in their correct sequence in the color circle. Of this type, two commonly used tests are the Farnsworth-Munsell 100-Hue and the Farnsworth Panel D-15 Test. As with PIPs, proper room lighting is necessary to obtain accurate results. The illumination used should approximate Standard Illumination "C," as established by the International Commission on Illumination. This illumination is best achieved with a Macbeth Illumina-

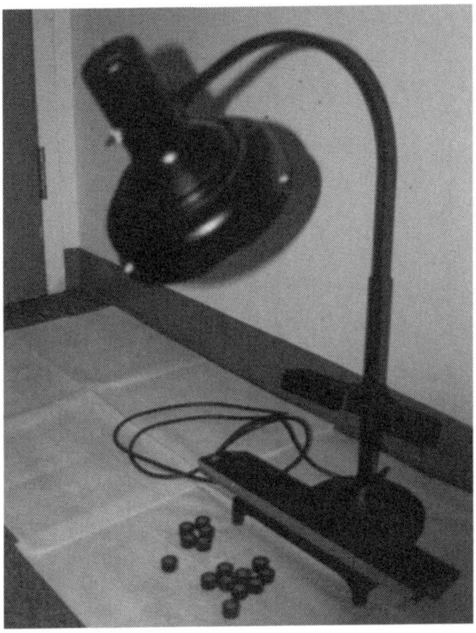

Figure 5.1
The Macbeth Illuminator provides Standard Illumination "C" as established by the International Commission on Illumination.

tor (Figure 5.1). It can also be approximated with ordinary daylight fluorescent lights or less accurately with natural daylight.

■ Farnsworth Panel D-15 Test

The D-15 consists of 15 movable caps that reflect 15 points along the color circle.[4] Proper illumination is necessary, and each eye is tested separately. The procedure for conducting the test is as follows:

1. The colored caps are placed in front of the patient in random fashion.
2. The patient is instructed to arrange the caps by placing the cap that looks most like the reference cap next to it. Next, the patient places the cap that looks the most like the one he or she just placed, and so on, until the sequence is complete. The caps can be rearranged if necessary.
3. On completion, the examiner inverts the caps by closing the box and turning it upside-down to reveal the concealed numbers underneath. The examiner records the sequence on the accompanying score sheet by drawing lines from number to number in the sequence chosen by the patient (Figure 5.2).

136 ☐ NEURO-OPHTHALMIC SYSTEM: CLINICAL PROCEDURES

FARNSWORTH DICHOTOMOUS TEST for Color Blindness—Panel D-15

Name...Age...5......Date....6/26/98......File No..............

Department...Tester.............................

DICHOTOMOUS ANALYSIS

Type	Axis of Confusion
PROTAN	(RED-bluegreen) ☐
DEUTAN	(GREEN-redpurple) ☐
TRITAN	(VIOLET-greenishyellow) ☐

PASS ☐
FAIL ☐

Test
Subject's Order 2 3 4 5 7 1 6 15 12 9 11 13 8 10 14
                 _ _ _ _ _ _ _ __ __ _ __ __ _ __ __

Retest
Subject's Order 1 2 3 4 5 6 7 8 15 9 10 11 12 13 14 15
Subject's Order 5 1 2 6 3 4 7 15 8 13 11 10 9 14 12
                 _ _ _ _ _ _ _ __ _ __ __ __ _ __ __

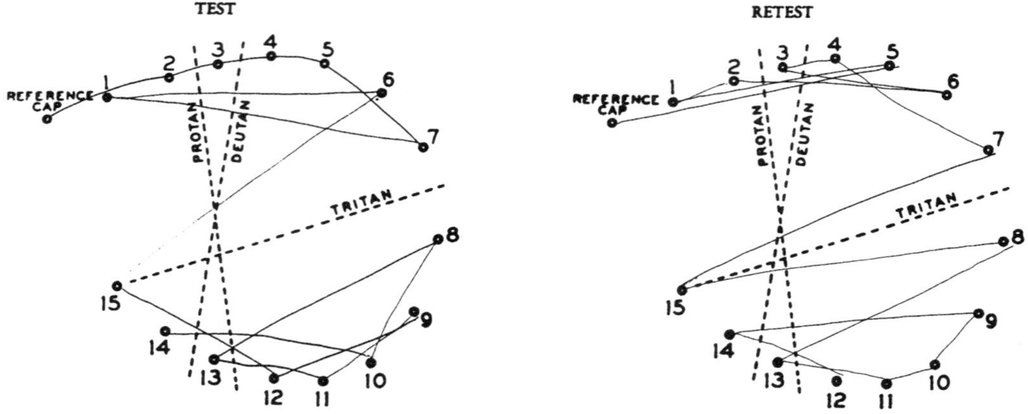

Figure 5.2
Results for the D-15 are recorded by drawing lines from number to number on the accompanying score sheet in the sequence shown by the patient. This example shows an acquired tritan defect.

Interpretation

If the numbers on the caps are not out of sequence, test results are normal. The lines corresponding to the sequence chosen by the patient will correspond to a reference pattern consistent with normal color vision or a congenital protan, deutan, or tritan defect. Acquired color vision defects will appear similar to congenital red-green or blue-yellow defects, but they will not appear as clean. Because the colors in the Panel D-15 are very saturated, the test is not sensitive enough to detect a low degree of acquired dyschromatopsia. Therefore, many patients with acquired color defects will pass. A variation of the test, Lanthony's Desaturated Panel D-15, is a less saturated version and therefore more useful in picking up mild, acquired dyschromatopsias.

■ Farnsworth-Munsell 100-Hue Test

The Farnsworth-Munsell 100-Hue test is an expanded version of the Panel D-15 test, consisting of 85 hues corresponding to 85 points along the color circle. It is very sensitive and is useful in determining the characteristics and severity of congenital and acquired color vision defects. The test contains four trays of colored caps, each with a fixed reference cap. Again, appropriate lighting is necessary to achieve accurate results. The procedure for conducting the test is as follows:

1. The colored caps from the first tray are placed in front of the patient in random fashion.
2. The patient arranges the caps in order, just as in the D-15. The same is repeated with the remaining three trays.
3. The cap sequence chosen by the patient is recorded on the accompanying score sheet just below the numbers corresponding to the correct sequence. Results are then transferred to the accompanying circular graph by combining the difference between the numbers of the caps to the right and left and adding the two numbers (Figure 5.3). For example, if the patient chooses a sequence of 1,3,4,2,6,5, the numbers on the circular graph would be 2,3,3,6,5, and so on.

Interpretation

The graph points are connected to form a diagram that has its highest error corresponding to a particular position on the color circle. The posi-

138 ☐ NEURO-OPHTHALMIC SYSTEM: CLINICAL PROCEDURES

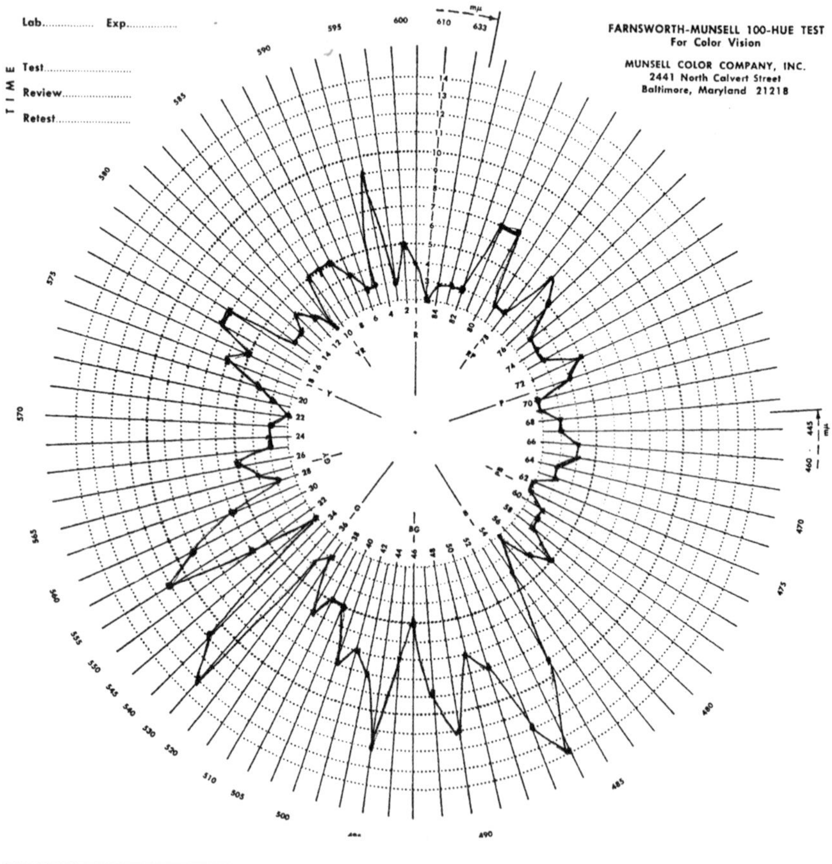

Figure 5.3 Results of the Farnsworth-Munsell 100-Hue test are recorded by combining the difference between the numbers of the caps to the right and left and adding them. The graph points are then connected to reflect the nature of the color vision loss. This is an example of a blue-green defect in a patient with mild ethambutol toxicity.

tion of the error will parallel a particular wavelength that reflects the nature of the color vision loss (see Figure 5.3). Scoring of this test is tedious and time-consuming, although it can also be scored by computer, making it a much more appealing test for the examiner.

■ Red Cap Test

Valuable information is often gained from a comparison of color saturation between the two eyes. This is particularly true of patients with acquired optic nerve disease where the color deficiency is more often asymmetric. In disease processes that affect the anterior visual pathway, color vision is often impaired before Snellen acuity is affected or may be disproportionately greater than impairment to achromatic stimuli.[5] The "red cap" test is therefore a useful adjunct to formal tests of color vision. The procedure for the red cap test is as follows:

1. The patient is seated in the examination chair and the room is fully illuminated.
2. A red target is presented monocularly at a distance of 40 cm. The patient is presented a red target monocularly to each eye and asked to compare the quality of the color between the two eyes. The first question is "What color do you see?" and on switching eyes, "Is it the same color or shade?"
3. If there is a difference, it can be qualified by presenting the target to the better eye and asking, "If the color is so good that it is worth $100, how much is it worth in the other eye?" Differences of $10 or less can usually be disregarded, whereas higher differences indicate a relative dyschromatopsia.

Interpretation

Patients with optic nerve disease will report that the color is "faded," "orange," "pink," "dim," or "brown" in the affected eye relative to the way it appears in the normal eye. The examiner must be sure that the patient does not misinterpret a blur from a refractive error or amblyopia as a true desaturation. A simple target (mydriatic cap), rather than a detailed target, is helpful in this respect. If the patient cannot detect a difference and the examiner is sure the question was understood, asymmetric optic nerve disease is highly unlikely. Red-green color vision is typically not affected with macular disease unless the extent is very severe[6] and easily seen clinically. Red desaturation is therefore not likely to be apparent in mild to moderate cases. It may, however, be noted with monocular or asymmetric lens changes.

Contrast Sensitivity

Contrast is defined as the degree of blackness to whiteness of a target.[7] Snellen acuity has long been the standard for determining the status of the visual system, and it measures the patient's ability to identify an object at maximum contrast. Although this has always been the standard for determining the status of the visual system, clinicians are too often faced with patients who have subjective complaints of visual disturbances despite normal Snellen acuity. Contrast sensitivity, for many years a test confined to research laboratories, has emerged as a more sensitive way of evaluating visual system function.

Contrast sensitivity is evaluated clinically by assessing the patient's ability to detect a bar grating at varying levels of contrast. Contrast sensitivity testing uses sine wave gratings, which have diffuse borders rather than square wave gratings that have sharply defined borders. By increasing the number of bars per degree of visual angle, contrast sensitivity can be plotted on a graph as a function of spatial frequency. The point at which the contrast sensitivity curve intersects the x-axis corresponds to the spatial frequency at which maximum contrast is needed to visualize the grating and is the equivalent of Snellen acuity. Snellen acuity therefore corresponds to just a single point on the contrast sensitivity curve and does not represent the whole spectrum of visual performance. From this, it is easy to conclude that overall contrast sensitivity can be reduced despite normal Snellen acuity. In fact, contrast sensitivity has been proven more sensitive than Snellen acuity in detecting visual system dysfunction.[8]

A number of commercially available tests of contrast sensitivity function are available to the clinician. The Vistech System (Vistech Consultants Inc., Dayton, OH) is the most widely used due to its relatively low cost, high accessibility, and simplicity. The VCTS 6500 is a 27-in. by 37-in. wall-mounted chart designed for use at a 10-m test distance. The chart contains five rows of nine sinusoidal grating patterns that are oriented vertically or tilted 15 degrees to the right or left of vertical. Spatial frequency increases from top to bottom, and the contrast level for each spatial frequency decreases from right

Additional Neuro-Ophthalmic Testing ☐ 141

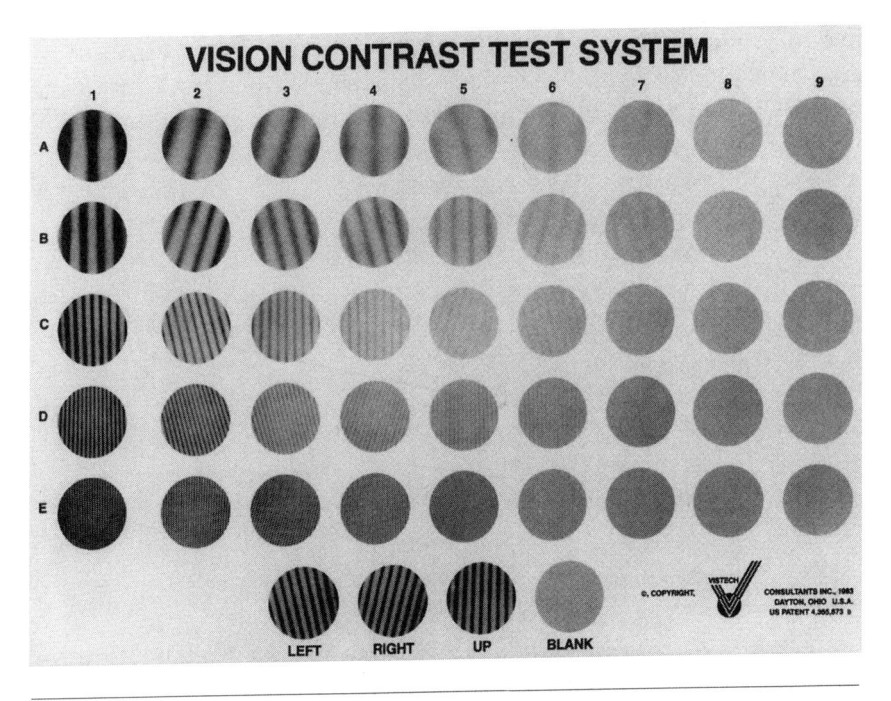

Figure 5.4 The Vistech 6500 contrast sensitivity system.

to left (Figure 5.4). The test is designed to measure contrast sensitivity under normal room lighting conditions so that light reflected off of the chart (luminance) should measure from 30 to 60 foot-lamberts. A light meter is included with the system so that appropriate lighting and standardization are possible. Vistech also has portable, near vision charts, a projection slide system, and an automated, tabletop system available for clinical use.

Contrast sensitivity testing with the Vistech 6500 is performed as follows:

1. The VCTS chart is placed at eye level and the patient is positioned at a test distance of 10 m.
2. Sample patches at the bottom of the chart with the three possible responses (left, right, or straight up) are shown to the patient.
3. One eye is covered with an occluder (the patient should not be allowed to use his or her hand to cover the eye because pressure on the eye may cause erroneous contrast sensitivity test results). Next, the patient is instructed to begin with row A and look across from left to right.

The patient is asked to identify the last patch in which lines can be seen and tell the examiner in which direction they tilt. If a response is incorrect, the patient should describe the preceding patch. The patient should then guess which way the lines tilt in the next patch. Guessing ensures the use of the three-alternative, forced-choice test method, known to improve the accuracy of contrast threshold measurement.

4. Each vertical column of numbers on the evaluation form corresponds to a horizontal row on the chart. The last patch the patient correctly identifies in each row is recorded by marking the corresponding dot on the evaluation form. Two different colors can be used to distinguish between the right and left eyes.

5. The marked points are connected to form a contrast sensitivity curve for each eye.

6. The other eye is now covered and the sequence repeated.

■ Interpretation

The patient's results are compared with the normal population range shown in the shaded area on the evaluation form (Figure 5.5). Contrast sensitivity curves have been investigated for a number of ocular disorders, including many of neuro-ophthalmic significance. Contrast sensitivity has been shown to equal the sensitivity of visual evoked potentials in patients with optic nerve disease and is more sensitive in detecting visual dysfunction in macular disease.[8] It has also been shown to be abnormal in patients with multiple sclerosis, compressive optic neuropathy, and cerebral lesions despite preservation of Snellen acuity.[9-11] In patients with recovered optic neuritis, subjective visual disturbances often persist despite recovery of Snellen acuity.[12] Contrast sensitivity in optic neuritis patients is abnormal in as many as 70% in either the medium- or both medium- and high-frequency ranges.[13] Contrast sensitivity has been shown to be useful in many other neuro-ophthalmic disorders despite normal Snellen acuity, including subclinical ethambutol toxic optic neu-

Figure 5.5 ► Contrast sensitivity results are recorded on accompanying score sheets, where they are plotted as a function of spatial frequency. This example shows reduced contrast sensitivity in the middle to high ranges in a patient with mild optic neuritis.

Additional Neuro-Ophthalmic Testing □ **143**

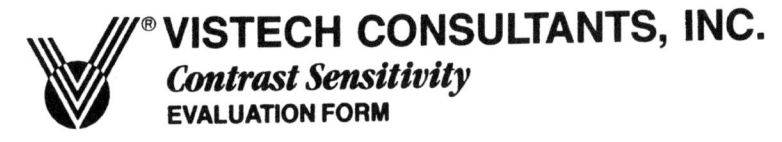

VISTECH CONSULTANTS, INC.
Contrast Sensitivity
EVALUATION FORM

CONTRAST SENSITIVITY / **CONTRAST THRESHOLD** vs **SPATIAL FREQUENCY (CYCLES PER DEGREE)**

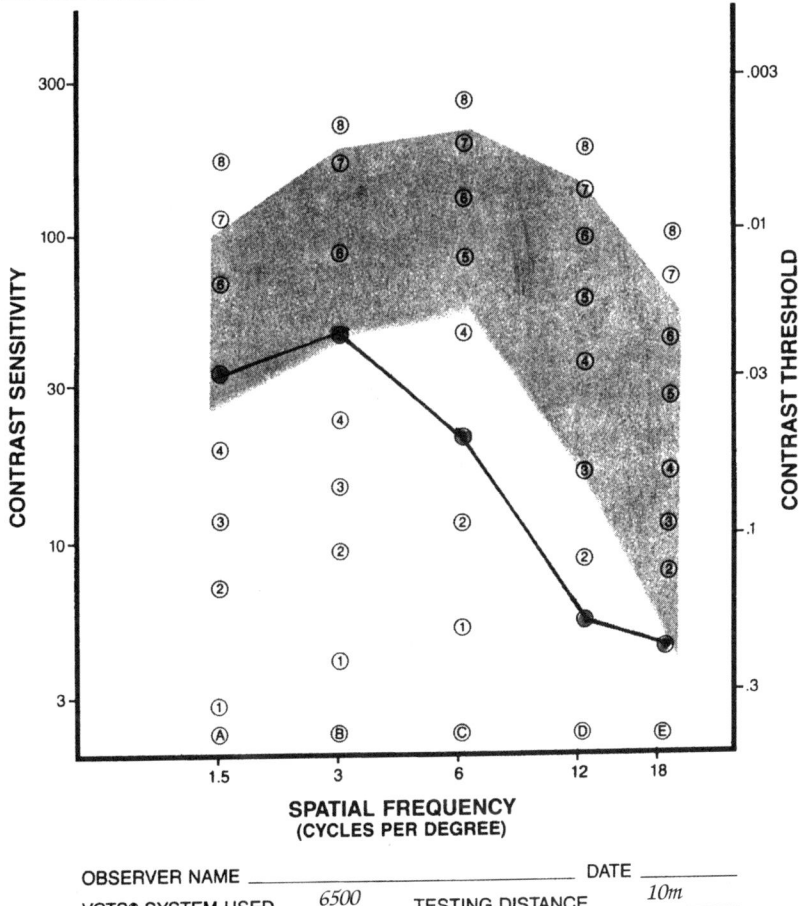

OBSERVER NAME _____ DATE _____

VCTS® SYSTEM USED __*6500*__ TESTING DISTANCE __*10m*__

COMMENTS: __*Optic Neuritis*__ _____

_____

Tested by: _____

The normal range of contrast sensitivity is shown in the gray area. The normal range is only relevant if proper lighting is used as described in the Instruction Booklet. It is provided to help AID in the diagnosis of optical, neurological, or pathological disorders and should not be used as a sole criterion for diagnosis and treatment. In some cases, depressed contrast sensitivity is due strictly to normal variation and not to an optical, neurological, or pathological problem. For this reason, contrast sensitivity should be used in conjunction with other diagnostic techniques.

ropathy,[14] Graves' optic neuropathy[15] (losses in the low-frequency range), and pseudotumor cerebri.[16]

Exophthalmometry

Exophthalmos is defined as an abnormal protrusion of the eyeball.[17] Exophthalmometry is the means by which such protrusion is measured. Documentation of exophthalmos is important because an eye that bulges abnormally may be harboring a vision- or life-threatening neoplasm, inflammatory disorder, or infection. Precise documentation of an exophthalmic state is important so that the clinician knows whether the causative condition is worsening and to help monitor the eye's response to treatment.

Detection of an exophthalmic state begins with careful inspection of the patient. In most patients, as little as 1–2 mm of asymmetric orbital protrusion is readily visible by simple inspection of the patient. This can be facilitated by leaning the patient backward or forward so that the globe position can be evaluated from above. When asymmetry is detected, the clinician must next identify the abnormal eye. Just as in cases where the eye bulges abnormally, an eye may sink back into the orbit (enophthalmos) as seen with orbital fractures with subsequent herniation of the orbital contents through a break in the orbital wall. Another important cause of enophthalmos is age-related shrinking of orbital fat with subsequent retrodisplacement of the globe. Careful history will help in the differential, and in the case of age-related enophthalmos, the eyes will appear sunken rather than protruding and the condition is usually bilateral and symmetric. An eye that appears to bulge forward should next be palpated by the examiner by placing the two thumbs or index fingers on the globe through closed eyes and gently retrodisplacing the globe (Figure 5.6). An eye that is pathologically exophthalmic will resist any attempt to retrodisplace it. On the other hand, an eye that easily retrodisplaces by approximately 2 mm is not likely to be harboring a neoplasm or other pathologic mass. In such cases, other causes should be explored to explain this pseudoexophthalmos, the most common etiology of which is high axial myopia. A refraction, followed by A-scan ultrasound, will confirm high axial myopia. Other causes of pseudoexophthalmos include asymmetric palpebral apertures, lid retraction, and anatomically shallow orbits.

A number of instruments are available to the optometrist for measurement of exophthalmos. Two popular instruments are the Hertel

Figure 5.6
Technique for retrodisplacing the globe.

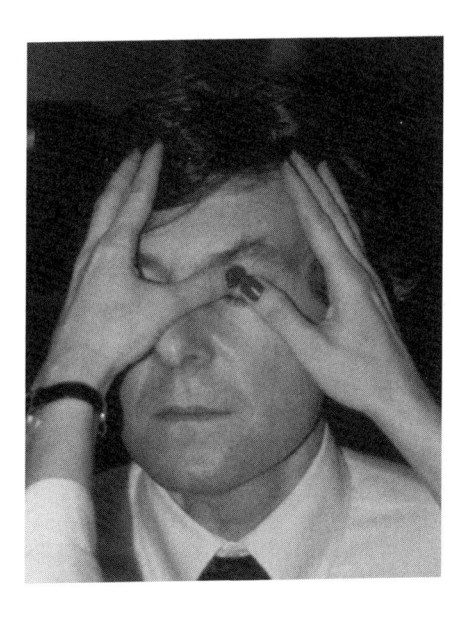

exophthalmometer and the Luedde exophthalmometer. Both are reputable instruments that are easy to use.

■ Hertel Exophthalmometer

The Hertel exophthalmometer[18] is perhaps the most widely used instrument for measuring globe displacement in clinical practice. It consists of a millimeter ruler with either a mirror or prismatic system that enables the examiner to view the lateral orbital rim and corneal apex in profile as if they were being viewed perpendicularly from the side. This makes it possible for the examiner to obtain lateral views on each side without moving.

The procedure for using the Hertel exophthalmometer is as follows:

1. The patient is seated and instructed to direct gaze straight ahead.
2. The examiner palpates the lateral orbital rim to locate the deepest point.
3. The set-screws of the instrument are loosened so that the width of the instrument can be adjusted. The foot plates of the instrument are then placed at each lateral orbital rim, and the screws are tightened (Figure 5.7). The reading on the crossbar is recorded as the base.

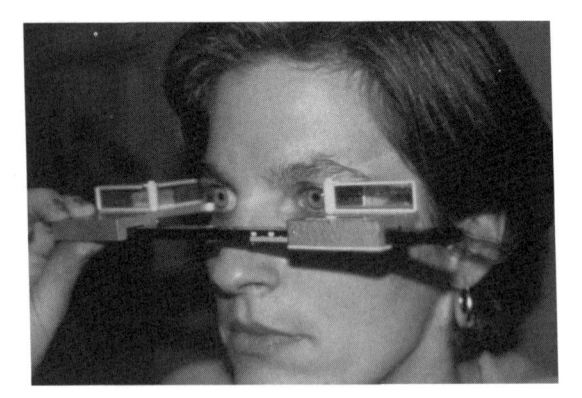

Figure 5.7
The Hertel exophthalmometer.

4. The examiner places his or her head directly in front of the patient's and adjusts his or her position so that the two red parallax lines are superimposed.

5. The marking on the ruler that is tangential to the corneal apex is recorded for both eyes, along with the base in the following manner:

$$\frac{18 \quad\quad 20}{110}$$

The reading above is 18 mm OD and 20 mm OS with a base of 110. The same base should be used for all future measurements for that patient.

If the mirrored version of the Hertel exophthalmometer is used, the procedure is the same except that there are no lines that correct for parallax before the measurement is obtained.

■ Luedde Exophthalmometer

The Luedde exophthalmometer[19] consists simply of a clear plastic square rod with a millimeter scale. The end is notched and tapered to fit snugly into the deepest part of the lateral orbital rim. The markings are placed on either side so that they can be superimposed when viewed from the side, minimizing parallax. The instrument is designed to be positioned perpendicularly to the plane of the face to ensure accurate readings; however, this can only be estimated by the examiner. A modified version of the device is available that connects two rods perpendicularly by a bar to

Figure 5.8
A modified version of the Luedde exophthalmometer consists of two measuring rods connected perpendicularly by a bar to facilitate accurate positioning.

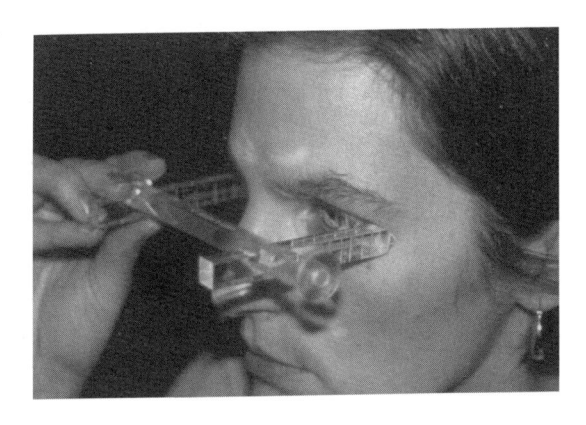

facilitate an accurate position (Figure 5.8). The procedure for using the Luedde exophthalmometer is as follows:

1. The patient is seated and instructed to direct gaze straight ahead.
2. The lateral orbital rim is palpated to locate its deepest point.
3. The notched end of the exophthalmometer is placed firmly into the deepest part of the lateral orbital rim while the examiner views the corneal apex from the side, at a position perpendicular to the sagittal plane through the apex of the cornea. The examiner's head position should be adjusted so that the notched markings on either side are aligned, eliminating parallax.
4. The device is positioned so that the apex of the cornea can be viewed and the point at which the apex of the cornea intersects the millimeter marking is recorded.
5. The sequence is repeated with the fellow eye.

■ Interpretation

Normal exophthalmometry readings vary by race, sex, and age. The normal upward limit is 20 mm for white women, 22 mm for white men, 23 mm for black women, and 25 mm for black men.[20] Between the ages of 10 and 18, readings increase by 3 mm.[21] Any difference between the two eyes of more than 2 mm is also suggestive of a pathologic process.

Carotid Auscultation

The carotid artery provides the vascular supply to the eye via the ophthalmic artery. Assessing the integrity of carotid blood flow is therefore an important aspect of the ocular health evaluation. The common carotid artery arises directly from the aorta on the left side and from the innominate artery on the right side. The extracranial carotid artery is easily accessible to the examiner by palpating the neck in the fleshy groove formed by the sternocleidomastoid muscle and cricoid cartilage. Carotid artery evaluation involves assessing the carotid pulse and auscultating for bruits. Occlusive disease of the carotid artery results in turbulent blood flow, which causes vibrations that are transmitted to the skin. The turbulence or bruit can be heard by placing a stethoscope on the skin overlying the carotid artery. Bruits typically have a low pitch, and the bell attachment of the stethoscope is best suited to hear them. On some occasions, however, bruits are accompanied by a higher pitch, which is better heard with the diaphragm attachment of the stethoscope.[22] The examiner should keep this in mind, especially when clinical suspicion is high and a bruit is not detected with the bell attachment.

The procedure for carotid auscultation is as follows:

1. The examiner locates the carotid artery by palpating in the fleshy groove created by the cricoid cartilage and the sternocleidomastoid muscle and feels for a pulse.

2. Beginning 1 inch above the clavicle, he or she places the bell attachment of the stethoscope on the neck and instructs the patient to stop breathing (Figure 5.9).

3. Moving upward along the course of the artery, toward the angle of the jaw, the examiner listens in three to four locations along the artery, each time instructing the patient not to breathe.

■ Interpretation

Occlusive disease of the carotid artery is most often due to atherosclerosis but can also occur from fibromuscular disease or vasculitis. The location and quality of the bruit provide useful clinical information.[23] Bruits heard in the supraclavicular area of the carotid artery can occur from aortic stenosis or carotid occlusive disease. In the former, the intensity tends to decrease

Figure 5.9
Carotid auscultation using the bell attachment of the stethoscope.

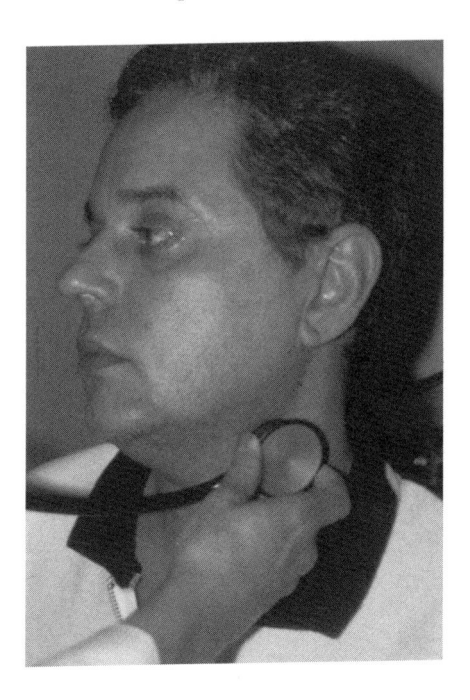

further up in the neck. Higher grade obstructive disease produces bruits of higher pitch and longer duration. Severely stenosed arteries are associated with faint murmurs; complete obstruction typically produces no bruit.

Orbital Auscultation

In much the same way the carotid arteries can be auscultated, the blood flow in the orbit can be assessed. Orbital bruits may be heard directly by placing the chest piece of the stethoscope over the globe or indirectly by placing it in bony areas around the orbit. The bruit may be more intense over the zygomatic and mastoid bones, where the diaphragm chest piece may be more effective.[24]

The procedure for orbital auscultation is as follows:

1. The patient is seated upright or lying supine.
2. The examiner places the chest piece of the stethoscope over the brow, zygomatic bone, maxillary bone, and mastoid processes (Figure 5.10).

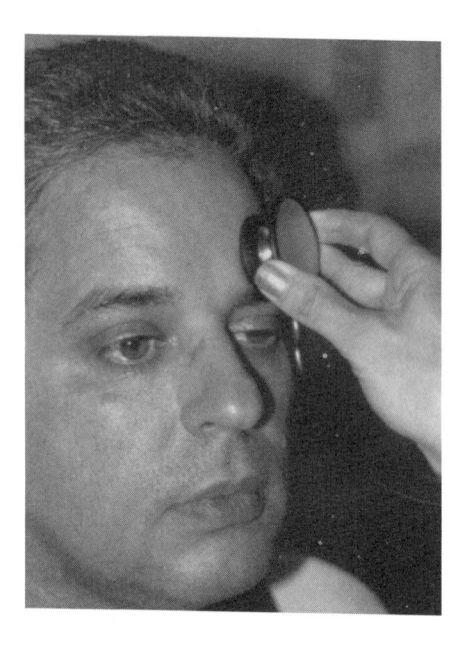

Figure 5.10
Orbital auscultation with the stethoscope positioned on the brow.

3. If a bruit is not heard, the globe is auscultated using the bell chest piece; the examiner should apply firm pressure through closed eyes.

■ Interpretation

An orbital bruit is typically associated with vascular lesions of the orbit such as arteriovenous fistulas and congenital vascular malformations.[24] Structural lesions of the orbit may alter blood flow, resulting in turbulence,[25] and carotid artery occlusive disease can result in a bruit that can be heard in or around the orbit.[26]

Ophthalmodynamometry

Ophthalmodynamometry (ODM) measures relative pressure in the ophthalmic artery. The ophthalmic artery is the first major branch of the internal carotid artery, and therefore, it reflects carotid circulation. The theory behind ODM is that if carotid artery perfusion is diminished due to occlusive disease, pressure in its branches will also be diminished. ODM involves applying external pressure to the eye while the arteries of the disc are observed. The resulting rise in intraocular pressure causes the arteries to pulse and then collapse. The point at which the vessel first begins to pulse corresponds to the diastolic pressure of the artery, and when the artery completely collapses, the systolic pressure is reflected.

The procedure for ODM is uncomplicated and requires simple equipment. Compression ODMs are more commonly used and are available in dial and linear models. The dial type has a round scale with two arrows: One actively moves with changes in pressure, and the other holds the position of the highest recorded pressure. The linear type has a hollow outer sleeve with a central post that has graduated markings. Pressure causes the outer sleeve to move along the scale.

Compression ODMs are more commonly used due to their relatively lower cost, but a number of difficulties have been encountered,[27] including the following:

1. The plunger must be held exactly perpendicular to the globe.
2. Friction of the piston against the lids, fingers, or mechanical stop.
3. Movement of the globe against the orbital contents may compress retrobulbar vessels.
4. Displacement of the globe with increased pressure from the instrument.
5. Abrasion of the cornea if the foot plate slips.

Suction ODMs are less commonly used because of their expense, but the difficulties encountered with compression ODMs are eliminated. Pressure is exerted on the globe by application of a vacuum.

Contraindications to ODM are unusual and include glaucoma, vascular occlusive disease, and any retinal disease that predisposes the patient to retinal detachment.[28]

Required equipment includes the ODM, ophthalmoscope, sphygmomanometer, stethoscope, mydriatic agents, and topical anesthetic.

The procedure for compression ODM is as follows:

1. The examiner dilates the patient's eyes with conventional mydriatic agents.

2. The examiner obtains brachial blood pressure readings from both arms.

3. When the patient is fully dilated, the examiner anesthetizes each eye.

4. The examiner provides a fixation target for the patient and places the foot plate tangentially on the temporal sclera approximately 1 cm from the limbus (Figure 5.11).

5. With the ophthalmoscope, the examiner locates an appropriate artery for observation on the optic disc and is careful not to mistake an artery for a vein, which will collapse at a much lower pressure. Use of a direct ophthalmoscope enables the examiner to work unassisted and provides better magnification; the use of a binocular indirect ophthalmoscope, although requiring an assistant, provides less magnification but a greater field of view.

6. The examiner gradually increases the pressure while directing the instrument toward the imaginary center of the globe. He or she should note the ODM reading when the artery first begins to pulse.

7. Once the first reading is noted, the examiner increases the pressure more rapidly until the vessel collapses. As soon as the vessel collapses, he or she notes the pressure and immediately removes the instrument from the eye. It is important to increase the pressure rapidly and remove the instrument immediately to avoid squeezing excessive fluid from the eye and altering intraocular pressure for successive measurements.

8. The measurements are repeated three times, with the examiner waiting 1 minute between each sequence. The examiner then eliminates any disparate readings and averages the results.

9. The results are then converted to millimeters of mercury (mm Hg) with the accompanying scale.

■ Interpretation

The diastolic arterial reading should be 45–60% of the diastolic brachial blood pressure, and the systolic reading should be 54–70% of the systolic brachial blood pressure. If the difference is greater, carotid occlusive disease is suggested on that side. Readings between the two eyes are compared as well. If the respective systolic and diastolic pressures differ by more than 20%, carotid occlusive disease is suspected on the side where pressure is lowest.

A more simplified interpretation of ODM results eliminates the need to compare brachial blood pressures with ODM readings.[29] The criteria

Additional Neuro-Ophthalmic Testing 153

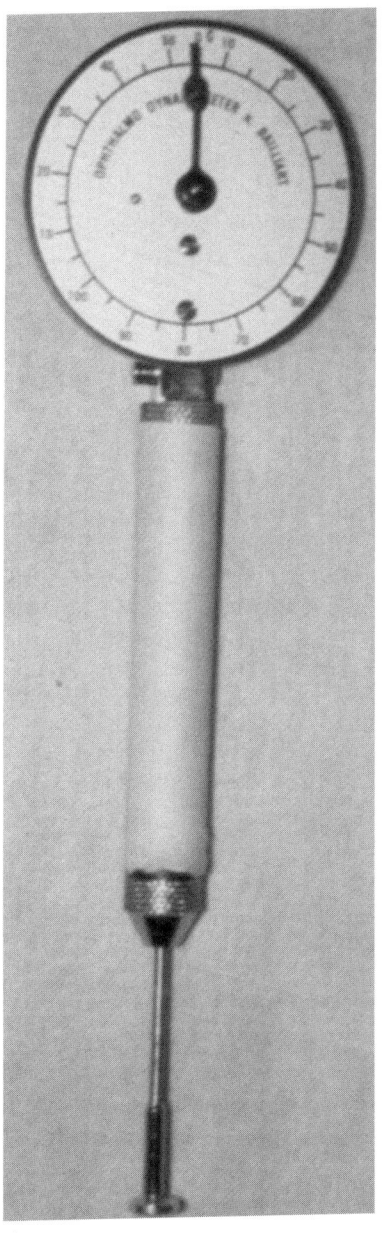

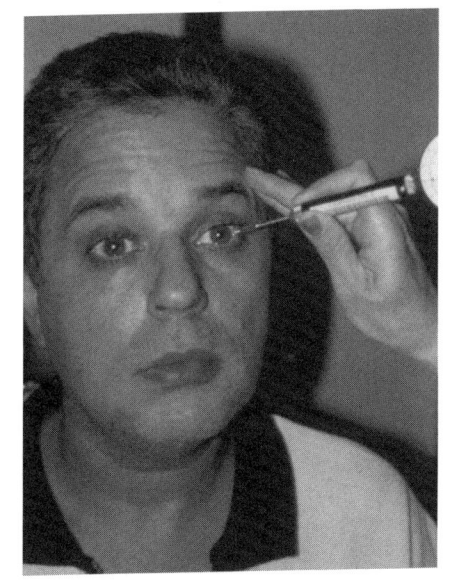

Figure 5.11
(A) Dial-type compression ophthalmodynamometry. (B) Placement of the instrument on the sclera.

used for an abnormal result are corrected systolic pressure of 70 mm Hg or less, a corrected diastolic pressure of 25 mm Hg or less, and a difference of 20% between the systolic or diastolic readings from the two sides. Using these criteria, ODM correctly identified carotid stenosis greater than 50% in 80% of the patients evaluated.[29]

Billing and Reimbursement

Specific billing codes apply to color vision testing and ODM. Contrast sensitivity, exophthalmometry, carotid auscultation, and orbital auscultation are not separate billable procedures, but they do support a higher level office code. The Current Procedural Terminology (CPT) code for color vision testing is 92283 and applies to PIPs, Panel D-15, and the FM 100 test. Testing with PIPs is considered to be part of an eye examination and cannot be billed separately. The CPT code for ODM is 92260.

Related International Classification of Diseases-9 (ICD-9) Terminology

Acquired color vision defect	368.55
Exophthalmos	376.30
Thyrotoxic exophthalmos	376.21
Amaurosis fugax	362.34
Central retinal artery occlusion	362.31
Branch retinal artery occlusion	362.32
Retinal ischemia	362.84
Hollenhorst plaque (partial retinal artery occlusion)	362.33

References

1. Kolner H. Die Storungen des Farbensines. Ihre Klinische Bedeutung und ihre Diagnose. Berlin: Karger, 1912.

2. Marre M, Pinckers A. Basic phenomena of acquired color vision defects. Bull Soc Belge Ophtalmol 1985;215:17–26.
3. Hardy LH, Rand G, Rittler MC. Tests for the detection and analysis of color-blindness. I. The Ishihara test: an evaluation. J Opt Soc Am 1995;35:268–275.
4. Farnsworth D. The Farnsworth Dichotomous Test for Color Blindness—Panel D-15. New York: Psychological Corporation, 1947.
5. Glaser JS. Clinical evaluation of optic nerve function. Trans Ophthal Soc UK 1976;96:359–362.
6. Verriest G. Further studies on acquired deficiency of color discrimination. J Opt Soc Am 1963;53:185–195.
7. Arden GG. The importance of measuring contrast sensitivity in cases of visual disturbance. Br J Ophthalmol 1978;62:198–209.
8. Skalka HW. Comparison of Snellen acuity, VER acuity and Arden grating scores in macular and optic nerve diseases. Br J Ophthalmol 1980;64:24–29.
9. Kupersmith MJ, Siegel IM, Carr RE. Subtle disturbances of vision with compressive lesions of the anterior visual pathway measured by contrast sensitivity. Ophthalmology 1982;89:68–72.
10. Kupersmith MJ, Nelson JI, Seiple WH, et al. The 20/20 eye in multiple sclerosis. Neurology 1983;33:1015–1020.
11. Bodis-Wollner I, Diamond SP. The measurement of spatial contrast sensitivity in cases of blurred vision associated with cerebral lesions. Brain 1976;99:695–710.
12. Trobe JD, Beck RW, Moke PS, Cleary PA. Contrast sensitivity and other vision tests in the Optic Neuritis Treatment Trial. Am J Ophthalmol 1996;121:547–553.
13. Fleishman JA, Beck RW, Linares OA, Klein JW. Deficits in visual function after resolution of optic neuritis. Ophthalmology 1987;94:1029–1035.
14. Salmon JF, Carmichael TR, Welsh NH. Use of contrast sensitivity measurement in the detection of subclinical ethambutol toxic optic neuropathy. Br J Ophthalmol 1987;71:192–196.
15. Suttorp-Schulten MSA, Tigssen R, Mourits MPH, Apkarian P. Contrast sensitivity function in Graves' ophthalmopathy and dysthyroid optic neuropathy. Br J Ophthalmol 1993;77:709–712.
16. Wall MW. Contrast sensitivity testing in pseudotumor cerebri. Ophthalmology 1996;93:4–7.
17. Taylor EG (ed). Dorland's Medical Dictionary (27th ed). Philadelphia: Saunders, 1988.
18. Hertel E. Ein einfaches exophthalmometer. Arch Ophthalmol 1905;60:171–175.
19. Leudde W. An improved transparent exophthalmometer. Am J Ophthalmol 1938;21:426.
20. Migliori ME, Gladstone GJ. Determination of the normal range of exophthalmometric values for black and white adults. Am J Ophthalmol 1984;98:438–442.
21. Fledelius H, Stubgard M. Changes in eye position during growth and adult life. Acta Ophthalmol 1986;64:481–486.

22. Carter SA. Arterial auscultation in peripheral vascular disease. JAMA 1981;246:1682–1686.
23. Hurst JW, Hopkins LC, Smith RB III. Noises in the neck. N Engl J Med 1980;302:862–863.
24. Glaser JS. Neuro-Ophthalmology (2nd ed). Philadelphia: Lippincott–Raven, 1990.
25. Cohen JH, Miller S. Eyeball bruits. N Engl J Med 1956;255:459–464.
26. Merritt HH. Neurological aspects of internal carotid obstruction. Bull NY Acad Med 1961;37:151–155.
27. Zaret CR, Sacks JG, Holm PW. Suction ophthalmodynamometry in the diagnosis of carotid stenosis. Ophthalmology 1979;86:1510–1512.
28. Toole JF, Wood FA. Carotid artery occlusion and its diagnosis by ophthalmodynamometry. JAMA 1957;165:1264–1269.
29. Mullie MA, Kirkham TH. Ophthalmodynamometry revisited. Can J Ophthalmol 1983;18:165–168.

Index

A

Abducens nerve, testing of, 115
Accessory nerve, testing of, 118, 119
Acoustic nerve, testing of, 117
Adie's tonic pupil, 55–56
   accommodative changes in, 56
   characteristics of, 56
   denervation (cholinergic) supersensitivity in, 56–57
   diminished corneal sensation in, 57–58
   diminished tendon reflexes in, 58
Afferent pupillary defect, 48–55
   grading of, 50–55
      with neutral-density filters, 51–54
      other clinical correlates and, 55
      with swinging flashlight test, 54–55
   swinging flashlight test for, 48–50. *See also* Swinging flashlight test
Afferent system disease, 44–45. *See also* Afferent pupillary defect
Amaurosis fugax, 130
Anisocoria. *See also* Pupillary function, evaluation of
   evaluation of, 39, 40–42
   physiologic, and swinging flashlight test, 49–50
Ankle jerk reflex, evaluation of, 127
Anterior ischemic optic neuropathy, and visual field defects, 87, 88–90
Argyll-Robertson pupil, 58

B

Babinski reflex (plantar response), evaluation of, 128
Balance, evaluation of, 124, 125–126
   Romberg test, 125–126
   tandem gait test, 125, 126
Biceps reflex, evaluation of, 127
Bielschowsky head-tilting test, 20–21
Biomicroscopy, 47

C

Carotid auscultation, 148–149
Cerebrovascular disease
   ocular manifestations of, 129–131
   risk factors for, 130, 131
Chiasmal disease, and visual field defects, 93–94, 95, 96
Cholinergic sensitivity, assessment of, 56–57
Cocaine, use of in diagnosis of Horner's syndrome, 61–62
Cochet-Bonnet esthesiometer, 57
Collier's sign, 58
Colobomas, optic nerve, and visual field defects, 92

Color vision testing, 133–140
  billing and reimbursement for, 154
  Farnsworth Panel D-15 Test, 135–137
  Farnsworth-Munsell 100-Hue Test, 137–139
  Macbeth Illuminator for, 134–135
  pseudoisochromatic plates, 133–134
  "Red Cap" test, 139–140
Confrontation visual field testing, 71–74
  comparison of colored targets, 73, 74
  finger counting, 72
  simultaneous finger counting, 72, 73
  simultaneous hand comparison, 72–73
Consensual response, 42, 44–45
Contrast sensitivity testing, 140–144
Coordination, evaluation of, 124–126
  finger-to-nose test, 124–125
  heel-to-shin test, 125
  rapid alternating hand and foot movements, 125
Corneal reflex test, 7, 8
Corneal sensitivity, assessment of, 57–58
Cranial nerve testing, 113–120
  CN I, 113–114
  CN II, 114–115
  CN III, IV, VI, 115
  CN V, 115–116
  CN VII, 116–117
  CN VIII, 117
  CN IX and X, 117–118
  CN XI, 118, 119
  CN XII, 118, 120
Cyclodeviations, measurement of with Maddox rod, 10, 12

D

Diplopia. See Strabismus, acquired, evaluation of
Dorsal midbrain syndrome, pupils in, 58
Drusen, optic nerve, and visual field defects, 92

E

Edrophonium (Tensilon) test for myasthenia gravis, 28–29
Esthesiometer, 57
Exophthalmometry, 144–147
  Hertel exophthalmometer for, 145–146
  Luedde exophthalmometer for, 146–147
Extremities, tests of, 121, 122
Eyelid, relationship of to pupil, 47

F

Facial nerve, testing of, 116–117
Farnsworth Panel D-15 Test, 135–137
Farnsworth-Munsell 100-Hue Test, 137–139
Finger-to-nose test for coordination, 124–125
Forced-duction test, 15–16
  with cotton-tipped applicator, 16
  with toothed forceps, 15–16
Fourth nerve palsy, 22–24

G

Glossopharyngeal nerve, testing of, 117–118
Goldmann perimetry. See Perimetry, manual
Graefe's sign, 26
Graves' ophthalmopathy, 24–26
  compressive optic neuropathy associated with, 26

eyelid retraction in, 26
mechanism of, 25
motility findings in, 25

H
Heel-to-shin test for coordination, 125
Hertel exophthalmometer, 145–146
Hirschberg test, 7
Horizontal misalignment, 2, 11, 17, 18, 19
Horner's syndrome, 41–42, 47, 59–64
  diagnosis of, 59–62
    dilation lag and, 60, 61
    inverse ptosis and, 59–60
    pharmacologic, 61–62
  localizing lesion in, 62–63
Hydroxyamphetamine, use of in localization of lesion in, 63
Hypoplasia, optic nerve, and visual field defects, 92

I
Internuclear ophthalmoplegia, 26–28

K
Knee jerk reflex, evaluation of, 127
Krimsky test, 7

L
Lancaster red-green test, 13–14
Lancaster screen, 6, 7
Lateral geniculate nucleus disease, and visual field defects, 97
Lesions, and vision field defects
  occipital lobe, 98, 100–105
  parietal lobe, 98, 99
  temporal lobe, 97
Levator function, testing of for myasthenia gravis, 30–31
Lower extremity drift, 121
Luedde exophthalmometer, 146–147

M
Macbeth Illuminator, for color vision tests, 134–135
Macular sparing, in occipital lobe disease, 100–101
Maddox rod, 6
Maddox rod test, 8–10, 11, 12
Medial longitudinal fasciculus, lesion of, 26–28
Mental status assessment, 112–113
  general information, 112
  interpretation, 113
  memory and concentration, 113
  orientation to time and place, 112
Midbrain disease, pupils in, 58
Motor examination, 120–122
Myasthenia gravis, 28–31
  diagnosis of, 28–30
    edrophonium (Tensilon) test for, 28–29
    sleep test for, 29–30
    testing of levator function and ptosis for, 30–31
    testing of orbicularis strength for, 31
  etiology of, 28
  ocular manifestations of, 28, 29

N
Near reflex, 37
Near response, 46
Nerves, testing of
  abducens, 115
  accessory, 118, 119
  acoustic, 117
  glossopharyngeal, 117–118
  oculomotor, 115
  optic, 114–115
  vagus, 117–118
Neurologic testing. *See* Systemic neurologic evaluation

Neuropathies, nutritional, and visual field defects, 85–86
Neutral-density filters,
  for diagnosing afferent pupillary defects, 51–53
  for grading of afferent pupillary defect, 51–54

O

Occipital lobe lesions, and visual field defects, 98, 100–105
Oculomotor nerve, testing of, 115
Olfactory nerve, testing of, 113–114
Ophthalmodynamometry, 150–154
  billing and reimbursement for, 154
Optic nerve,
  colobomas, and visual field defects, 92
  disease, color vision in, 133
  drusen, and visual field defects, 92
  hypoplasia, and visual field defects, 92
  testing of, 114–115
Optic neuritis, and visual field defects, 86
Optic tract disease, and visual field defects, 95–96
Orbicularis strength, testing of for myasthenia gravis, 31
Orbital auscultation, 149–150

P

Pain sensation, evaluation of, 123
Palsies
  fourth nerve, 22–24
  sixth nerve, 24
  third nerve, 21–22
    pupil in, 64
Parietal lobe lesions, and visual field defects, 98, 99, 100
Parinaud's syndrome, pupils in, 58

Parks Three-Step Test, 18–21
Perimetry
  automated, 81–84
    disadvantages of, 82
    Humphrey's STATPAC and, 82–83
  with chiasmal disease, 94
  manual, 74–79
  and neuro-ophthalmic visual field defects, 75–80
  procedure for, 74–75, 76, 77
Postchiasmal pathway disease, and visual field defects, 94–104
Prism and cover test, 8, 9
Proprioception and position sensation, 124
Pseudoisochromatic plates, in color vision testing, 133–134
Pseudotumor cerebri, and visual field defects, 87–88, 91
Pupil gauge, 41
Pupillary function, evaluation of, 35–47. *See also* Pupils, disorders of
  anatomy, 35–38
  history taking, 38–39, 40
  materials for, 39–40
  tests for, 40–47
    biomicroscopy, 47
    direct and consensual response, 42, 44–45
      swinging flashlight test, 44. *See also* Swinging flashlight test
    eyelid position, 47
    measuring pupil sizes in bright and dim illumination, 40–42
    near response and pupillary light–near dissociation, 46
    pharmacologic, 47
Pupillary light reflex, parasympathetic control of, 35–36

Pupillary light–near dissociation, 46
Pupillary pathway, sympathetic control of, 37–38
Pupils, disorders of, 48–65. *See also* Pupillary function, evaluation of
 afferent pupillary defect, 48–55. *See also* Afferent pupillary defect
 billing and reimbursement for, 65–66
 Horner's syndrome, 59–64. *See also* Horner's syndrome
 in midbrain disease, 58
 from pharmacologic blockade, 65
 third nerve palsy, 64
 tonic, 55–58
  Adie's (idiopathic), 55–58. *See also* Adie's tonic pupil
  local, 55
  neuropathic, 55

R
Red lens, 6
Red lens test, 10–11, 13
Reflexes, evaluation of, 127–128
 ankle jerk, 127
 Babinski (plantar response), 128
 biceps, 127
 knee jerk, 127
 triceps, 127
Riddoch phenomenon, 77
Romberg test for balance, 125, 126

S
Sella turcica, and chiasmal disease, 93–94
Sensory evaluation, 122–124
 light touch, 124
 pain, 122–123
 proprioception and position, 124
 temperature, 123

Sixth nerve palsy, 24
Skew deviation, 28
Sleep test for myasthenia gravis, 29–30
Strabismus, acquired, evaluation of, 1–33
 age of patient and, 5
 billing and reimbursement for, 32
 history taking, 1–7
 identification of paretic muscles in, 17–21
  horizontal misalignment and, 17, 18, 19
  vertical misalignment and, 17–21
  Parks Three-Step Test for, 18–21
 interpretation of, 21–31
  fourth nerve palsy, 22–24
  Graves' ophthalmopathy, 24–26. *See also* Graves' ophthalmopathy
  internuclear ophthalmoplegia, 26–28
  myasthenia gravis, 28–31. *See also* Myasthenia gravis
  sixth nerve palsy, 24
  third nerve palsy, 21–22
 materials for, 5–7
 tests for, 7–16
  corneal reflex, 7, 8
  forced duction, 15–16
  Lancaster red-green, 13–14
  Maddox rod, 8–10, 11, 12
  prism and cover, 8, 9
  red lens, 10–11, 13
Stroke
 ocular manifestations of, 129–131
 risk factors for, 130, 131
Sweating patterns, and localization of lesion in Horner's syndrome, 63, 64

Swinging flashlight test, 44, 48–50
  sources of error in
    indirect afferent pupillary defect, 50
    physiologic anisocoria, 49–50
    physiologic hippus or pupillary unrest, 49
    stimulus intensity, 48–49
    test speed, 49
Sylvian aqueduct syndrome, pupils in, 58
Systemic neurologic evaluation, 111–132
  billing and reimbursement for, 131
  with cerebrovascular disease and stroke, 129–131
  coordination and balance, 124–126. *See also* Balance, evaluation of; Coordination, evaluation of
  cranial nerve testing, 113–120. *See also* Cranial nerve testing
  indications for, 111
  mental status assessment, 112–113. *See also* Mental status assessment
  motor examination, 120–122
  reflexes, evaluation of, 127–128. *See also* Reflexes, evaluation of
  sensory evaluation, 122–124. *See also* Sensory evaluation

T
Tandem gait test for balance, 125, 126
Tangent screen visual field testing, 80–81
Temperature sensation, evaluation of, 123
Temporal crescent, preservation of in occipital lobe disease, 101–104

Temporal lobe lesions, and visual field defects, 97
Tensilon test for myasthenia gravis, 28–29
Third nerve palsy, 21–22
  pupil in, 64
Tilted discs, and visual field defects, 92
Tobacco/alcohol neuropathies, 85–86
Tonic pupil. *See* Pupils, disorders of, tonic
Touch, light, evaluation of sensation of, 124
Toxic neuropathies, and visual field defects, 85–86
Transient ischemic attacks, 130
Triceps reflex, evaluation of, 127
Trigeminal nerve, testing of, 115–116
Trochlear nerve, testing of, 115

U
Upper extremity drift, 121

V
Vagus nerve, testing of, 117–118
Vertical misalignment, 2, 3, 17–21
Vistech System for testing contrast sensitivity, 140–144
Visual field
  defects of
    in chiasmal disease, 93–94, 95, 96
    in congenital optic nerve anomalies, 91–93
    functional, 104, 106
    neuro-ophthalmic, Goldmann approach to, 75–80
      Riddoch phenomenon, 77
    in nonglaucomatous optic nerve disease, 84–87
      anterior ischemic optic neuropathy, 87, 88–90

optic neuritis, 86
pseudotumor cerebri, 87
toxic and nutritional, 85–86
in postchiasmal pathway disease, 94–104
  lateral geniculate body, 97
  occipital lobe lesions, 98, 100–105
  optic tract disease, 95–96
  parietal lobe lesions, 98, 99, 100
  temporal lobe lesions, 97
definition of, 70–71
evaluation of, 69–110
with automated perimetry, 81–84. *See also* Perimetry, automated
billing and reimbursement for, 107–108
with confrontation testing, 71–74. *See also* Confrontation visual field testing
identification of patients for, 69–70
with manual perimetry, 74–79. *See also* Perimetry, manual
purpose of, 69
with tangent screen, 80–81